The Medicine You Take

D. R. LAURENCE, MD, FRCP, qualified in medicine in 1945. He has spent his professional career in the University of London, and is now professor of Pharmacology and Therapeutics at the School of Medicine, University College, London.

He has been particularly concerned with the design and conduct of investigations of drugs in man and has worked largely with drugs acting on the cardiovascular and nervous systems. He served on the UK drug regulatory organization (Committee on Safety of Medicines) for 14 years, and is now a member of the Medicines Commission. He is author of a text-book, *Clinical Pharmacology*, now in its fourth edition.

J. W. BLACK, FRCP, FRS, qualified in medicine in 1946. He has worked in the Universities of St Andrews, Glasgow and London where he was (until recently) Professor of Pharmacology at University College. He has also had 15 years of industrial research experience, working particularly on drugs acting on hormone receptors in the heart (beta-adrenoceptor blockers) and in the stomach (histamine H_2-receptor blockers). He has recently taken up an appointment as Director of Therapeutic Research with the Wellcome Foundation Ltd (UK).

TECHNOSPHERE

Technosphere is a series that presents individual studies of particular sciences and technologies in terms of their human repercussions. The series will include original analyses of a wide variety of subjects with the emphasis in each case on the present state of the science or technology in question, its social significance, and the future direction of its probable and necessary development.

The series editor is Jonathan Benthall, author of *Science and Technology in Art Today* and *The Body Electric: Patterns of Western Industrial Culture*, editor of *Ecology: The Shaping Enquiry* and *The Limits of Human Nature*, and co-editor of *The Body as a Medium of Expression*. Formerly lecture programme organizer at the Institute of Contemporary Arts, he is now Director of the Royal Anthropological Institute.

Already published

Alternative Technology and the Politics of Technical Change
David Dickson

Television: Technology and Cultural Form
Raymond Williams

D. R. Laurence and J. W. Black

The Medicine You Take

Benefits and risks of modern drugs

Fontana Paperbacks

First published in Fontana 1978

Made and printed in Great Britain by
William Collins Sons & Co Ltd Glasgow

Contents

Preface

This book is about the problems of providing relief of human suffering safely and effectively by means of drugs. It ranges from technical pharmacology to politics, and from general statements about populations to highly personal individual experiences. At the end we offer our conclusions.

Modern technological medicine is nowadays much criticized for waiting for disease to occur and then trying to cure it rather than seeking to prevent it from occurring in the first place. It is also criticized for failure, as judged by population health statistics.

It is pointed out, for example, that improved living conditions, rather than medical treatment, has played the major role in the enormous decline in the death rate from infectious diseases over the past 100 years. It is true that the biggest changes in some important areas of health result from social and economic developments rather than from the application of technical medicine. And 'prevention is better than cure' is a familiar saying because it is true.

But people still frequently fall sick and will continue to do so, although the pattern of disease in the community changes, infectious disease in the young giving place to degenerative disease in the old. We must look at population statistics; but we must also, in a humane society, look to the individual sufferer.

It is good to prevent tuberculosis; but those few, in rich countries, as well as the many in poor countries awaiting the arrival of preventive measures (higher living standards), who are yet unfortunate enough to contract the disease, will be grateful for drugs.

It is good to prevent cancer, and ways of doing so for some cancers, e.g. stopping smoking, are known, though seldom adopted; but those who fall sick will be grateful for drugs, surgery and radiation, whether these cure or only ease the passage through the last phase of life.

It is better to prevent some heart disease, by moderate and

sensible living, including moderation in eating, though such measures are all too little adopted; but those who fall sick will be grateful for drugs.

It would be better, if we only knew how, to prevent rheumatoid arthritis, epilepsy, pernicious anaemia, many cancers, and diabetes, but we do not know how, and sufferers are grateful for drugs. This list could be prolonged indefinitely.

It is not our intention in this book to argue the case for relative investment of resources, money and skills, in preventive medicine and in curative medicine. This book is about one important aspect of technological medicine, drugs, which are used both to cure and to prevent sickness.

Modern science and technology have put many tools into man's hands. The car, the aeroplane, electricity, cheap books, are all in themselves neither good nor evil. But they are potent and can be used with either result. Which it will be is in the hands of the users.

Most drugs in common use in orthodox medicine are also products of modern science. Properly used their benefits are enormous, though, as with the aeroplane and electricity, there are inherent risks due to their very nature, as well as to the innate capacity for error of human beings.

It may be the case that drug science has grown faster than the public and the health professions have learned to use its offerings. It is therefore necessary to make a special effort to win the enormous benefits of modern drugs whilst avoiding their risks. This end will be achieved by increased understanding and knowledge of drugs not only in the health professions but amongst the public. But there must be a willingness to be educated and informed.

This book is about drugs, their benefits, risks, actions, discovery, control and use. The authors are professionals in drug science and between us we have 60 years full-time research and education in the field.

It is our intention to help people to understand drugs better so that they can not only participate more effectively in the continuing public debate on cost and 'whither medicine', but so that they can know more or less what they can reasonably expect from drugs when they themselves fall sick, and ask their doctor, 'Isn't there something you can give me to make me better?' The sufferer hopes the answer will be 'yes' and is unlikely to be comforted by being told that his condition could, and perhaps even should, have been prevented. Indeed many patients would be offended by such a reply, even when it is true; they want relief, and they want it now.

We have included some relatively technical aspects of drug science because we believe that the most specialized topics can be explained using a minimum of technical jargon (the convenience of the professional) and that minimum can be explained in the text or in a glossary. Readers who are not interested in following these technical accounts may skip them without losing the thread of the book.

We hope the book may be interesting to the public in general, but particularly to young people contemplating a career in biological, chemical or medical sciences.

We are grateful to our friends who, knowingly and unknowingly, have contributed to this book; we especially thank Rosalind Pitt-Rivers and John Maddox. We also thank the authors and publishers who have allowed us to quote from their works.

D. R. LAURENCE
J. W. BLACK

NOTES

1. The royalties from the sale of this book are being applied to research and training in Clinical Pharmacology at the School of Medicine, University College, London.

2. Parts of this book appear in *Clinical Pharmacology* by D. R. Laurence and P. N. Bennett (Churchill Livingstone).

1. Balancing benefits and risks

'Somewhere between 1910 and 1912 in this country . . . a random patient, with a random disease, consulting a doctor chosen at random had for the first time in the history of mankind, a better than fifty-fifty chance of profiting from the encounter.'[1]

Everybody knows that drugs[2] can do good.

Medically this good may sometimes be trivial, as in the avoidance of a sleepless night in a noisy hotel or of social embarrassment from a profusely running nose due to seasonal pollen allergy (hay-fever). Even such benefits, however, are not necessarily trivial to the recipient, concerned to be at his best in urgent matters, whether of business, pleasure or passion.

Or the good may be literally life-saving, as in the prevention of death from serious acute infections (pneumonia, septicaemia) or in the prevention of life-destroying disability from severe asthma, from epilepsy or from blindness due to glaucoma.

Everybody knows that drugs can also do harm.

This harm may be relatively trivial as in hangover from a hypnotic or sleepiness from an antihistamine used for hay-fever (though these may be a cause of serious road accidents).

The harm may also be life-destroying as in the rare sudden death following an injection of penicillin, rightly regarded

[1] Attributed to Lawrence Henderson, biochemist, Harvard University (USA) (New Engl. J. Med. 1977. *296*, 448).

[2] A *drug* is a single chemical substance that forms the active ingredient of a *medicine*, which latter may contain many other substances to deliver the drug in a stable form acceptable and convenient to the patient. The terms will be used more or less interchangeably in this book. To use the word 'drug' intending only a harmful, dangerous or addictive substance is to abuse a respectable and useful word.

as one of the safest of all antibiotics, or the slower death or disability that occasionally attends the use of drugs that are highly effective in asthma and rheumatoid arthritis.

Everybody, the patient, the physician and the developer of new drugs (who is almost always employed in profit-making industry) wants effective and safe drugs or medicines[2] just as everybody wants effective and safe food and transport.

There are risks in taking medicines just as there are risks in food and transport. There are also risks in not taking medicines when they are needed, just as there are risks in not taking food or in not using transport when they are needed.

In all these areas both public and private endeavour should be devoted to maximizing benefit and minimizing harm. Much is being done in the field of drugs as well as in those of food and transport. More could be done. It is not only necessary to have good drug scientists (pharmacologists) and technologists working on the problems, but also good social scientists, good politicians and good businessmen and good administrators. These requirements are more likely to be fulfilled if the public is well informed and understands what can and what cannot be reasonably expected of drugs. Then the public can bring pressure to bear to implement sensible policies, moderating the pressures of extremists and fanatics.

Efficacy and safety do not lie solely in the chemical nature of a drug. Doctors must choose which drugs to use, and must do so usually in an increasingly complicated field. Then patients must use the prescribed medicine correctly. For self-medication it is necessary to have proper promotion, labelling and instructions, and the user should pay attention to these. In addition, success or failure of drug therapy may be influenced by the patient's apprecation of his position and his willingness to co-operate (patient 'compliance' or 'adherence'); this particularly applies when assiduous attention is required from both doctor and patient over many years, as in the management of epilepsy, diabetes or high blood pressure, where the patient may feel well but understands the need to maintain an inconvenient therapy to remain well.

The patient, whether suffering or merely inconvenienced, expects drugs to relieve him; the doctor wishes to meet this expectation. From the moment when the doctor is faced with the patient, practical problems begin; should a drug be used at all, and if so, what is the ratio of benefit to risk?

The great physician Sir William Osler[3] wrote in 1894: 'But know also, man has an inborn craving for medicine . . . The desire to take medicine is one feature that distinguishes man the animal from his fellow creatures. It is really one of the most serious difficulties with which we have to contend.'

And it is indeed so: the patient wanting relief; the doctor wishing to provide it; and the drug manufacturer wishing, like any other commercial enterprise, to sell as much as he can. The pressures to ask for, to provide and to consume are great, and all would be well (except for expense)[4] if drugs were entirely safe. But they are not entirely safe. A person who uses drugs or who allows them to be administered undertakes, whether he knows it or not, a risk, just as he does when he uses electricity or gas in his home, eats, drinks, or travels; in each case much of the risk is contributed by people or factors over whom or which he has no control except indirectly and partially through government.

That there are risks in taking drugs is often remembered, but that there are also risks in not taking drugs is often forgotten. This latter, even when not forgotten, is sometimes given less prominence than it deserves. It is easier to count the number of thalidomide babies than it is to quantify the suffering that goes unrelieved when an effective drug is not prescribed or is not available. People naturally take a different view of risks they think they can understand from risks they cannot understand or evaluate. The risks of drugs are commonly in the latter class; they are further discussed in Chapter 3.

People holding strong views in one direction have tended to stress the undoubted horrors of some drug accidents, and this is understandable when the most notorious accident involved a hypnotic drug (thalidomide) for which there were numerous alternatives and that was often used for trivial reasons. Those holding strong views in the other direction have sometimes seemed callous in their assertion that requirements for safety-testing in animals may become excessive

[3] Sir William Osler (1849-1919), successively Professor of Medicine in the Universities of McGill (Canada), Philadelphia (USA), Johns Hopkins (USA), Oxford (UK).

[4] Not all drugs are expensive: many life-saving drugs are cheap.

and inhibit the development of useful new drugs.

We hope, by discussing drugs and medicines, how they work, what can reasonably be expected of them, what risks may be considered acceptable, to provide an account that will be of interest to all who have used drugs (and who has not?) as well as an introductory account to those who are considering making a special study of these fascinating, useful, hazardous substances.

Note: a glossary of technical terms will be found at the end of the book, though many are also defined in the text.

2. Assessing the benefits

'For those who did not enter medical practice until the end of the 1930s, it is difficult to imagine the devastating uncertainty in life produced by lobar pneumonia,' writes Sir Harold Himsworth.[1]

'It came like a bolt from the blue, attacking all ages indiscriminately. A fit man in the prime of life, with a wife and young children dependent on him, would go to work feeling perfectly well. In the middle of the afternoon, he would be seized with a headache. An hour or so later, he would be feeling so ill that he would have to go home. A week, sometimes only 48 hours, later he would be dead. In different epidemics the mortality rate ranged from 5 to 20%. And there was nothing, apart from giving, at most, marginal help, that we could do for our patients save to try and sustain their strength until the crisis occurred in a week or ten days' time.

'In the Spring of 1937 or 1938, we were experiencing a bad epidemic. In hospital, where the more serious cases were, we were losing one patient in four; and I was getting desperate. But I had heard rumours about a new drug called M & B 693 (the code number given to sulphapyridine by its industrial developer, May and Baker) and I was fortunate enough to get hold of an advance supply. As soon as it arrived I dashed up to my wards (where I had a dozen patients, in five of whom the outlook was grim) and told my house physician to give the drug straight away. Next morning, when I came to hospital, he was waiting on the front steps, hardly able to contain himself. He grabbed my arm and said I must come to the wards at once. I went with a sinking

[1] Sir Harold Himsworth, FRS (1905-), lately Physician and Professor of Medicine, University College Hospital, London and Secretary, Medical Research Council (UK). Personal communication.

heart. There he took me from patient to patient. All the temperatures were normal. All were sitting up in bed sparkling. I could not believe my eyes, for we were seeing something that no human being had ever seen before. That was the end, for all practical purposes, of what Sir William Osler called "the captain of the men of death",[2] lobar pneumonia.

'Ten years later, a young man with this condition was admitted into one of my beds. After I had examined him, my house physician asked if he could go back and listen to his chest again. He did. He then turned to me and said, "Do you realize, this is the first case of lobar pneumonia I have seen in my life?" By then, of course, they were all being treated at home, for with modern treatment, ordinary lobar pneumonia has become little more serious than a severe cold.'

This is a dramatic example of curative drug therapy. But not all therapy is curative. *Drugs are used in three principal ways:*
1. *curative:* as primary or ancillary (auxiliary) therapy.
2. *suppressive:* of disease or of symptoms.
3. *preventive.*

A few examples only will be given and they will be of two kinds:
(a) uncontroversial, where we believe any reasonable person who took the time and trouble to study the available evidence would reach the same conclusion.
(b) controversial, where issues of great importance to the patient are involved and it is, quite simply, hard to reach a consensus because of the difficulty and complexity of the subject.

1. CURATIVE

In the use of curative drugs a notable area of success is that of bacterial and parasitic infections. Here drugs are frequently life-saving or reduce what would have been a severe and/or prolonged illness to a mere inconvenience.

[2] A phrase originally used of tuberculosis by John Milton (1608-74).

A personal experience of *lobar pneumonia* (affecting one of the 2/3 lobes of the lung) is described above. The 1935 revision of the famous text-book of medicine written by Sir William Osler said:

'As a rule, the disease sets in abruptly with a severe chill, which lasts from fifteen to thirty minutes or longer. In no acute disease is an initial chill so constant or so severe. The patient may be taken abruptly in the midst of his work or awaken out of sleep in a rigor. The temperature during the chill shows that the fever has already begun. If seen shortly after the onset, the patient usually has features of an acute fever and complains of headache and general pains. Within a few hours there is pain in the side, often agonizing; a short, dry, painful cough begins, and the respirations are increased in frequency. When seen on the second or third day, the picture in typical pneumonia is more distinctive than in any other acute disease. The patient lies often on the affected side; the face is flushed, particularly one or both cheeks; the breathing is hurried, accompanied often with a short expiratory grunt; the [nostrils] dilate with each inspiration; . . . the eyes are bright, the pupils are often unequal, the expression is anxious, and there is a frequent short cough which makes the patient wince and hold his side. The expectoration may be blood-tinged . . . After persisting for seven to ten days if a crisis occurs, with the fall in temperature the patient passes from a condition of extreme distress and anxiety to one of comparative comfort.'

In 1935 the sulphonamides (synthetic antibacterial drugs) were introduced.[3] In one study in which 100 patients were treated with the new drug, which itself was not free from risks, the mortality was 8% whilst in 100 patients managed concurrently according to the best standard treatment it remained at nearly 30%. This convincing evidence led to the general acceptance that sulphonamides saved lives in pneumonia. A few years later penicillin was introduced and has remained the drug of choice up to the present.

Lobar pneumonia in a previously healthy person no longer

[3] By G. Domagk (1895-   ), a scientist working in industry in Germany.

carries the distress and risk that it did, with the anxious wait for up to 10 days for the 'crisis' when the fever dropped dramatically as the immune responses of the body at last killed the invading bacteria. With penicillin about half the patients have a normal temperature within 12 to 36 hours and the remainder within 4 days.

For several years before the introduction of modern chemotherapy for *tuberculosis* in the 1940s the decline of death rate from the disease had been 3% a year. With the introduction of effective drugs this annual reduction in the death rate suddenly improved to 15% a year, and by 1960 the rate was less than one-tenth that of 1940. Whilst general hygiene and improved standards of living have greatly, though slowly, influenced the *incidence* of the disease, they do not explain the dramatic changes in death rate. Current studies in developing countries also dramatically confirm the benefits of drugs to those who have already acquired the disease.

'Among the achievements of chemotherapy in this disease three in particular deserve mention. It has enabled patients with advanced disease to be rendered fit for surgery. It has saved many lives from tuberculous meningitis, which formerly was invariably fatal. Last, but not least, it is capable of rendering almost all patients sputum-negative,[4] thereby eliminating risk to their contacts and removing the need for sanatorium treatment.'[5]

Syphilis, spread by sexual contact, was probably never cured at all before 1906 though the older treatments with the toxic metals mercury and bismuth may have modified its course. So serious is the disease that it was justifiable to use toxic arsenic compounds initially when research in artificially infected animals predicted their efficacy as cures. But these have been superseded by penicillin to which drug the causative spirochaete is always sensitive. The effective treatment of syphilis has relieved untold suffering in those who

[4] i.e. living, and so infective, bacteria are no longer present in the spit; a person who previously had to be isolated in a sanatorium may now remain at home without risk to spouse and children.

[5] Garrod, L. P. (1970), *British Medical Bulletin*, 26, 187.

contracted it from sexual intercourse as well as protecting the children born to mothers with the disease. The 'sins' of the parents need no longer be visited on the children.

As well as being the prime *cure* of some diseases, drugs are often important, and even essential, *ancillaries* to the treatment of disease.

The best example is *anaesthesia*, whether it be the local anaesthetic that reduces routine dentistry from an ordeal almost to mere boredom or the general anaesthesia that allows the leisurely and careful surgery of hernias, appendicitis, abnormalities of the heart, organ transplants and the reparative procedures necessary after motor accidents. The adventurous and skilled surgeon becomes a public figure but, as he will readily acknowledge, it is the often anonymous and highly skilled anaesthetist with his drugs who renders the surgeon's work possible.

We are aware nowadays that the use of drugs poses social, religious and moral as well as merely technical problems, and, when passions rise over the use of oral contraceptives, it may be salutary to reflect that such current disputes may one day be regarded with the kind of wry humour with which we can now look back on the nineteenth-century religious objections to anaesthesia as being unnatural and against the will of God.

'Dr Simpson [the discoverer of chloroform] refers, in his pamphlet on the religious objections which have been urged to chloroform, to the first operation ever performed — namely the extraction of the rib of Adam, as having been executed while our primogenitor was in a state of sopor, which the professor learnedly argues was similar to the anaesthesia of chloroform. He further draws a justification of his own proceedings from the history of the creation of man. Putting aside the impiety of making Jehovah an operating surgeon, and the absurdity of suggesting that anaesthesia would be necessary in His hands, Dr Simpson surely forgets that the deep sleep of Adam took place before the introduction of pain into the world during his state of innocence.'[6]

Another field where drugs are ancillary is obstetrics

[6] *Lancet* (1848), *1*, 292.

(though pregnancy and childbirth are not diseases in the ordinary sense, it is convenient to include them here).

The use of drugs to relieve pain in *childbirth* was, similarly, in the early nineteenth century considered by some to be immoral as interfering with God's will that women should suffer. This extreme moral view was probably only ever held by a vocal and fanatical male minority, and it soon subsided; but obstetric analgesia has been a matter of technical controversy since 1853 when, as the *Lancet* recorded: .

'A very extraordinary report has obtained general circulation connected with the recent accouchement of her most gracious Majesty Queen Victoria. It has always been understood by the profession that the births of the Royal children in all instances have been unattended by any peculiar or untoward circumstances. Intense astonishment, therefore, has been excited throughout the profession by the rumour that her Majesty during her last labour was placed under the influence of chloroform, an agent which has unquestionably caused instantaneous death in a considerable number of cases. Doubts on this subject cannot exist. In several of the fatal examples persons in their usual health expired while the process of inhalation was proceeding, and the deplorable catastrophes were clearly and indisputably referrible to the poisonous action of chloroform, and to that cause alone.

'These facts being perfectly well known to the medical world, we could not imagine that any one had incurred the awful responsibility of advising the administration of chloroform to her Majesty during a perfectly natural labour with a seventh child. On enquiry, therefore, we were not at all surprised to learn that in her late confinement the Queen was not rendered insensible by chloroform or by any other anaesthetic agent. We state this with feelings of the highest satisfaction. In no case could it be justifiable to administer chloroform in perfectly ordinary labour; but the responsibility of advocating such a proceeding in the case of the Sovereign of these realms would, indeed, be tremendous. Probably some officious meddlers about the Court so far overruled her Majesty's responsible professional advisers as to lead to the pretence of administering chloroform, but we believe the obstetric physicians to whose ability the safety of our illustrious Queen is confided do not sanction the use of chloroform in natural labour. Let it not be supposed that we would undervalue the immense importance of chloroform in surgical operations. We know that an incalculable amount of agony is averted by its employment. On thousands of occasions it has been given without injury, but inasmuch as it has destroyed life in a considerable number of instances, its unnecessary inhalation involves, in our opinion, an amount of responsibility which words cannot adequately describe.

'We have felt irresistibly impelled to make the foregoing observations, fearing the consequences of allowing such a rumour respecting a dangerous practice in one of our national palaces to pass unrefuted. Royal examples are followed with extraordinary readiness by a certain class of society in this country.'

In fact the Queen did receive what she described in her private Journal as 'that blessed chloroform', adding that 'the effect was soothing, quieting and delightful beyond measure'.[7]

Pain-free labour sometimes occurs spontaneously and no doubt may be promoted by appropriate psychological and physical preparation for the event, but, rightly or wrongly, most women, in Western civilizations at least, anticipate pain and demand relief. The reasons that there still remain differences of opinion on how to achieve relief are that the medical requirements are stringent and much depends on the skill with which the drugs are used. The ideal drug must relieve pain without making the patient confused or unco-operative; it must not interfere with uterine activity, nor must it influence the fetus adversely, particularly the initiation of breathing immediately after delivery. The drug must also be safe and effective in the hands of a midwife without specialist medical supervision.

Immediately after the delivery of the placenta it is important that the uterus should contract to prevent bleeding from the site of its attachment to the uterine wall; this site has a profuse supply of blood vessels because its function is to provide from the mother all that the fetus needs for growth and development. Normally the uterus contracts spontaneously at this stage, but if it does not do so serious and even

[7] Quoted by C. Woodham-Smith: *Queen Victoria*: Hamish Hamilton, London. 1972.

fatal bleeding can occur. It has become routine practice to give a drug (ergometrine, ergonovine or sometimes oxytocin) at this point to eliminate the risk. Only rarely does the drug cause any adverse effects and these are trivial compared with its benefits.

Even more controversial is the use of oxytocin (in fact a purified natural hormone from the pituitary gland or a synthetic form of this) to start a woman in labour and to control the speed of labour. There is general agreement that in a minority of cases the onset of labour may naturally be so much delayed as to constitute a hazard to the fetus, and in such cases intervention, including the use of drugs, is beneficial. But since the means to start and control labour are available their use has spread beyond these uncontroversial cases to situations of special convenience of the patient and even of the doctor. This spread was encouraged by the increasing use of a specialized anaesthetic technique (epidural anaesthesia) involving insertion of a tube into the lower spinal column; the technique gave a painless labour but required expert supervision that is more easily available during ordinary working hours.

In one centre in the UK in 1974 the number of cases in which labour was artificially induced had risen to 56% of patients; in 1976 the figure had fallen to 25%. Changes of such magnitude in management of what is generally a normal process suggest that this practice came into such extensive use without comprehensive evaluation of all its implications. In this case there is little doubt that public anxiety was a factor causing obstetricians to review their practice.

Induction and control of labour with drugs provide an example of the complex consideration, technical, psychological and social that surround the use of drugs in many areas.

The above exemplifies the use of drugs for primary care of disease (bacterial infections), as ancillaries to cure by another means (surgery) and to facilitate an essential function (childbirth).

2. TO SUPPRESS DISEASES AND SYMPTOMS

Suppression comprises the continuous or intermittent use of drugs to maintain health without attaining cure, i.e. when drug therapy stops, the disease process, which was always present, though its manifestations were suppressed, manifests itself again. Sometimes the disease may regress because it is self-limiting so that continuation of therapy becomes unnecessary; sometimes the disease itself is intermittent. Although it must always be a second best to curative drug therapy, suppressive therapy is useful in a wide range of diseases.

Examples include high blood pressure, diabetes mellitus, peptic ulcer, rheumatoid arthritis, asthma, epilepsy, some mental disorders.

If the *blood pressure* is sufficiently high for a long period it has been convincingly shown that life is shortened owing to effects on brain, heart and kidneys. In the most severe cases (malignant hypertension), before effective treatment became available in the 1950s, 90% of patients died within a year of diagnosis; the new drugs immediately halved this mortality. In less severe cases there has been a substantial reduction in complications affecting brain, heart and kidneys. In the mildest cases, without symptoms, and which are usually detected by chance when the blood pressure is measured during a routine medical examination for employment or insurance purposes, it is by no means certain that treatment is necessary. Large studies are in progress to determine whether or not many symptom-free people should be encouraged or even persuaded to take drugs for many years.

In *peptic ulcer*, sufferers have often discovered for themselves, before they ever see a doctor, that antacids (stomach powders, indigestion remedies) rapidly provide effective though short-lived relief of pain. But they do not generally cause the ulcer to heal. Drugs that actually increase healing are either only marginally effective (carbenoxolone, Biogastrone) or are still too recently developed (cimetidine, Tagamet) for their true place to be defined.

In *rheumatoid arthritis* drug therapy is of substantial value. It relieves much pain and stiffness and allows many, especially younger, people to lead an active life which the untreated disease would otherwise prevent. But adverse reactions to the drugs used are comparatively common. In advanced cases actual destruction of the smooth joint surfaces by disease has taken place and drugs cannot, of course, restore these.

In *asthma* numerous sufferers attest for themselves that their lives are transformed by effective drug therapy, and the same is true of *epilepsy*.

Synthetic or natural hormones are used to replace deficiencies when these occur as a result of disease of the natural endocrine tissues. Important examples include failure of pancreatic secretion of insulin (diabetes mellitus), of thyroid secretion (hypothyroidism), of the adrenal cortex (Addison's disease), of the lining of the stomach (pernicious anaemia). In all these cases the untreated patient will either die or become an invalid. Effective treatment restores him to what amounts to normal life and in some cases (pernicious anaemia) the expectation of life even becomes normal, but only provided treatment is maintained for life.

In the case of *diabetes mellitus* it is the form with an onset in early life (juvenile form) that is due to deficiency of insulin and that is treated by replacement of insulin; in the form with an onset in middle life (maturity-onset form), often accompanied by obesity, it is the tissues that fail to respond to insulin produced by the pancreas rather than deficient production of insulin; this form is treated differently, by synthetic drugs (if the patient is not restored by appropriate diet and by reduction of weight) the effects of which over years remain uncertain and controversial.

The use of drugs in *mental disorders* is widespread but is relatively controversial compared with the general agreement that exists in regard to diseases such as high blood pressure or epilepsy.

A reasonably open-minded investigator might be expected to conclude from an examination of the evidence that drugs such as the phenothiazine tranquillizers (chlorpromazine, Largactil) contributed substantially to the management of acute schizophrenic episodes but that the benefits of these drugs in long-term management of chronic schizophrenia required much more study before a definitive conclusion could be reached.

In acute depression, drugs, particularly of the important tricyclic group (imipramine, Tofranil), are probably effective and may prevent many suicides. Plainly the use of the words 'probably' and 'may' in the previous sentence greatly weakens its claim. Evaluation of drugs in conditions where non-drug factors are a major influence on the course of the disorders, as is commonly the case in psychiatry, is peculiarly difficult. Some of the problems of drug evaluation will be discussed in a later chapter.

In anxiety, again, it is in the acute cases that benefits of drugs are most readily seen; long-term use in chronic anxiety remains a much more dubious matter.

Few who have studied the matter will deny that drugs have a valuable part to play in the management of mental disorders, that many will consider that this part is secondary to other measures, and that perhaps most will agree that, in our present state of ignorance, there is much uncritical though well-intentioned overprescribing of drugs for these conditions.

Suppression of symptoms of disease, i.e. pain, cough, insomnia, travellers' diarrhoea, is an area of drug therapy familiar to anyone likely to read this book. For such purposes, drugs, sensibly used, are a boon, despite the fact that all of them can have effects that nobody wants, i.e. their use entails risk, though usually a very small risk.

3. TO PREVENT DISEASE

Drugs may sometimes be valuable to prevent us from contracting a disease we have not got, but to which we are or will be exposed.

Examples include:

Malaria: when a non-immune person enters a malarial area he needs to take a drug to protect his health and indeed his life; this practice is normally highly effective, but drug-resistant parasites occur.

Travellers' diarrhoea is a familiar condition, particularly in certain parts of the world indicated by some of its popular names, the Aztec two-step, Montezuma's Revenge, Delhi Belly, Gyppy Tummy, Hong Kong Dog, Rangoon Runs, Casablanca Crud and Estomac Anglais. The Mexican name for it, *turista*, indicates a principal group of sufferers in our restless society. There are probably several causes, of which bacterial infection is only one. Although the disease is normally self-limiting (1-3 days) it is extremely unpleasant and can also be socially embarrassing.

Optimists take a wide variety of drugs to prevent it.

The balance of evidence is that prevention is ineffective and that early treatment by drugs that constipate, e.g. codeine phosphate or diphenoxylate plus atropine (Lomotil) is the wisest course. The benefits of that modern folk-remedy Entero-Vioform (clioquinol) are dubious and in large doses there is risk of serious damage to the brain and spinal cord, an outbreak of which has occurred in Japan.

The largest-scale use of drugs for prevention is in *contraception* (though pregnancy is not strictly a disease). Here the efficacy and therefore the benefit is in no doubt whatever. The principal medical issue for debate is the occurrence of adverse effects, chiefly blood clotting (thrombosis) that can, though rarely, be fatal. At present the balance of opinion lies heavily that for most women the undoubted benefits outweigh the undoubted risks, and this is an area where the patient or consumer, adequately informed, may expect to make the decision for herself. The patient alone knows the importance to herself of effective protection against pregnancy and she can legitimately expect her doctor to advise her of the potential risks (which vary with her past medical history and her age).

But when it comes to the detail of the choice of one preparation from among the many (about 30 in the UK) available, then the patient is unlikely to want any detailed discussion and will generally expect the doctor to have the technical knowledge to choose the drug for her, just as in the choice of drug for high blood pressure, depression or rheumatism the doctor is expected to prescribe what will suit the patient best without going into technical details as to whether, as in the case of hypertension, the drug should be guanethidine, bethanidine, guanoxan, guanoclor, debrisoquine, methyldopa, reserpine, hydrallazine, propranolol, sotalol, metoprolol, timolol, clonidine, prazosin, chlorothiazide, hydrochlorothiazide, bendrofluazide, methyclothiazide, etc. Sometimes, as in some forms of combination of drugs for cancer or general anaesthesia (where ten or more drugs may be used for one operation), any involvement of the patient in choice of drugs is hardly practicable.

Decision-taking is a process that, depending on the circumstances, may or should be made largely by the patient, largely by the doctor or any balance of sharing in between. There is a danger that doctors, exercising a paternalism that is unintentionally arrogant, may sometimes usurp the right of the patient to take personal decisions, especially those involving the acceptance of risk.

General statements based on accumulated evidence of efficacy such as have been made hitherto may suffice to impress healthy people who are both imaginative and acquainted with disease. But many of the healthy have difficulty in appreciating the impact of diseases on the life of sufferers as well as the bliss that effective treatment can bring.

The following descriptions of disease and personal accounts from sufferers (for sources see end of chapter) are included to help bring home to the healthy what it is really like to be sick and to help the healthy to understand why the sick are so often willing to take risks to obtain relief; that to be offered a choice of relief though with risk is better than to wait for the far-off day, if indeed it should ever come, when relief can be offered without any risk.

We are in no doubt that if we suffered from any of the diseases listed below we would be prepared to take risks to realize even a remote hope of succour.

Pernicious anaemia is a condition in which the body is unable to absorb vitamin B_{12} from food. Lack of vitamin B_{12} results in a fatal incapacity to form red blood cells. Vitamin B_{12} is stored in the liver; in 1926 it was discovered that injections of extracts from animal liver cured the anaemia; in 1948 the pure vitamin was isolated and this is now used instead of liver extract. For a fatal disease there has been substituted the minor nuisance of a small injection every third month.

'My name is Ted and in 1928 I applied for a job on the railway as a maintenance joiner, this being my trade. My age then was 27, and after a medical examination – I was passed **A1** – I began work in the engineer's department. Sometimes, with bridge repairs and so on, it was hard going, but I was in good health and never bothered about the weather.

'The war came, and by 1940 everyone was working at top speed. We were at it ten hours a day for seven days a week; I was also assigned as captain of the rescue party and secretary of the fire-watching party, and was carrying on with trade-union business. After three years of this I began to feel a bit tired, so I went to my doctor, who gave me a fortnight's convalescence. Again the next year, 1944, I began to feel the strain, so I applied for a transfer to the motive-power department. Still I felt more and more tired; and that year I spent my fortnight's leave at home.

'Returning to work, I ran into real trouble, with pain in the head coming on about noon each day, and backache somewhere round the kidneys, which made it hard to sit still with any comfort. I tried all kinds of remedies and did get a little relief for short periods from aspirin and backache pills . . . My doctor told me that overwork was the cause of the trouble; and when I had heard this from him two or three times I stopped going to the surgery.

'Then, in 1946, I began to lose my temper very quickly; and I felt that I did not want anyone to bother me at all. If I had not been a good servant in the past and had not had a good supervisor, I think my services would have been no longer required.

'So we come to 1947. One day I sat down to do some thinking, and I thought to myself, "Now, Ted, you'll have to shake this thing off"; but it was easier said than done. Each day I cycled six miles to work; and this was a strain. I was very bad-tempered, and if approached by any of my mates I would be very sarcastic; and I was always in trouble with someone. My wife must have the patience of Job. All I wanted to do was sleep, and the more I slept the more sleep I wanted. I still carried on, hoping to improve, but I did not. At the beginning of 1948 I could not ride my bicycle up any kind of incline: I seemed to be short of breath and my heart would beat like a steam-hammer working overtime . . . the worst trouble was that I didn't feel like working, and nothing seemed to go right. I would start a job, but something always went wrong; then I would throw it aside in disgust and sit down; being alone in the workshop I was fast asleep in a minute or two, and woke up only when an engine came past.

'About this time my mates began to tell me I looked . . . yellow . . . so in May I took a holiday in Holland. The first day after I got back I set out for work, but had to stop. I just felt like entering into the gates of heaven; so I returned home the best way I could think of. The next day I went to hospital, anxious to know what was going to happen. The doctor asked me how I felt, and I replied "fed up". He examined me from top to toe and then told me I was suffering from pernicious anaemia. This was the first shock; the second came when he told me I should have to stay a month in hospital. Having never been in hospital before, my one thought was to get home.

'The rest is quickly told. A week after the injections were started I began to feel better; and two weeks' convalescence at the seaside got rid of the rest of the weakness. Now, with regular injections of liver extract, I feel as good as ever I did. In fact, I haven't really got what you would call a disability. The only thing is that if I'm a bit late with an injection I somehow feel the need of it; so I try to keep on time.'

Epilepsy is a disease of recurrent convulsions. As well as physical hazard it has major emotional and social implications for the sufferer. In about 75% of epileptics drugs eliminate the fits altogether or else reduce their frequency; despite this achievement a lot of suffering continues unrelieved.

A medical sufferer writes:

'Epilepsy is defined in the dictionary as the "falling sickness". I do not propose to enter into an academic discussion concerning types, characteristics, and causation of such seizures; I will tell quite simply what happens if I have a fit.

'It starts with a peculiar sensation in my chest, but before I can do anything about it I am unconscious. I know and feel nothing. On recovery, I have a feeling of extraordinary well-being: wherever I happen to be lying, whether on a couch, the floor, or even the roadside, it is as if I were lying on the most comfortable bed. I may hear voices asking if someone has injured herself and I wonder of whom they are talking. If I notice someone looking down at me with evident concern, I wonder at the anxiety shown. After a few seconds,

I am completely awake; I find that I am lying on the floor, remember the aura,[8] and know that I must have had another fit. I feel myself gingerly to make sure that I'm whole, get up, and that is all.

'That is my version of the event, but what do spectators think? Perhaps I have been talking to them a few moments previously, I utter a cry and fall to the floor. My arms and legs jerk convulsively, my lips are covered with saliva, and my breathing is stertorous. After a very short interval these movements cease and I lie still, but my face remains pale and my eyes are open and appear vacant. It is a shock to whoever is present; they feel baffled and helpless. They wish to help, but there is little to be done: the interval during which I lie inert seems interminable, and because there is nothing much they can do their imagination becomes active. The person with me wonders what would have happened if the fit had occurred a few moments earlier when I might have been with a patient, or an hour later when I might have been alighting from a bus in a busy street, and determines that I must not run such risks in future.

'These two opposing viewpoints magnify the difficulties which we epileptics have to overcome.'

A nurse writes:

'. . . of the barrier which exists between the epileptic and the non-epileptic. There was an implication that there was no future in nursing for me, and that I had been guilty of a grave misdemeanour in having hidden my handicap. Although, in my new post, I met with kindness and consideration from the medical officers under whom I worked, I cannot describe the mental anguish which I suffered. It is better to forget this period; it was dominated by feelings of frustration, guilt, fear, and loneliness. For two years I was "unstable", but then I began to adopt a more reasonable attitude. I realized that if as an epileptic one cannot do the work of one's choice one must make the best of the work one is allowed to do, and interest in it will develop.

'Besides making adjustments to the work one can reason-

---

[8] Premonitory sensation, often an 'uneasy feeling' in the upper abdomen.

ably be allowed to do, one must learn to live with people who do not want to have the embarrassment of an epileptic thrust on them in their leisure hours. To do my job I must live away from home. I find the best way of managing is to take a furnished room and be independent of outside help. It is often wiser to keep one's secret, and to move to other rooms if trouble arises with the landlady; although sometimes an unexpectedly helpful attitude is shown. Household tasks – cooking, cleaning, mending, and shopping – occupy several evenings usefully and happily. An occasional meal in a restaurant, a visit to a cinema or theatre, provide diversion. The natural anxiety which my parents felt for my safety had to be allayed. My own powers of persuasion proved inadequate, but they agreed with my views more readily after reading some of the booklets published by the American League Against Epilepsy.

'The solution of such problems is an individual matter, but epileptics who have met with much social frustration would welcome the advice of a social worker. I realize that the rather placid life which appeals to me, a woman of 40, would not satisfy an adolescent. I have talked to many epileptics, some of them young men and women on the threshold of life, eager for companionship and adventure. I have been impressed with their good sense, and their desire to help each other. Perhaps the social problem could be solved by the formation of an association for epileptics;[9] such an association would help us to learn more about each other, and would teach us that we face a common difficulty. It would serve an excellent purpose if it became the channel through which the simple truth about the condition could be made known to the general public.'

Another writes:

'Others find it hard to understand the epileptic's difficulties. As a sufferer from grand mal I have found that broadly these are threefold.

'First, nobody is entirely "master of his fate", but the normally healthy person can both think and behave as if he were. For the epileptic this is impossible. The feeling that

[9] The British Epilepsy Association was founded in 1951.

at any moment with no chance of escape, he can have his life blacked out, his whole pattern of living interrupted, can be at times – and particularly just after an attack – quite terrifying. Even if he can overcome this feeling he has to behave as though nothing which he does or plans is certain. It is so easy to come to regard life as a mere matter of existing, and nothing more.

'Secondly, there is the feeling of resentment. I suppose that this is a feature of most long-term afflictions, yet I believe that it must affect epileptics more than most. Just because, between attacks, there is no outward sign, just because one's disability is what one might call an "invisible wooden leg", it is almost impossible to get other people to accept one's limitations at their true value. It is bad enough to think of all the things that might have been but cannot be, in the matter of jobs and other activities, without feeling that one must lose still more because an employer, or one's own sense of fairness, decides to play safe.

'Thirdly, there is the attitude of others to epilepsy as a disease. It is not so much the fact that by its nature it discourages sympathy except in those who come into close contact with it. It is the quite positive attitude among those who are ill-informed – and how many they are – that epilepsy is a "little bit queer" and faintly repulsive.'

It is plain that even better drugs are needed and this means more research. In epilepsy even a minor improvement in efficacy that benefits a few patients is likely to be considered a blessing by those few, and it should not be dismissed as 'mere molecular manipulation'. It is possible to be over-critical of minor variants of drugs.

Myasthenia gravis is an uncommon disease in which there is a defect in the transmission of the nerve impulse to voluntary muscle so that although an initial movement may be normal, repeated movements rapidly become weak and the patient may be unable to co-ordinate the eyes, walk, or in severe cases, even breathe.

The sudden appearance of an effective treatment for a hitherto untreatable chronic disease must always be a dramatic event for its victims. The impact of the discovery of the action of neostigmine has been described by one patient. Neostigmine prevents the normally rapid destruction of the chemical transmitter (acetylcholine) released at the endings of nerves that supply the muscles, thus intensifying its effect.

'My myasthenia started in 1925, when I was 18. For several months it consisted of double-vision and fatigue . . . An ophthalmic surgeon . . . prescribed glasses with a prism. Soon, however, more alarming symptoms began.' Her limbs became weak and she 'was sent to an eminent neurologist. This was a horrible experience. He . . . could find no physical signs . . . declared me to be suffering from hysteria and asked me what was on my mind. When I answered, truthfully, that nothing was except anxiety over my symptoms, he replied, "My dear child, I am not a perfect fool . . ." and showed me out.' She became worse, and at times she was unable to turn over in bed. Eating and even speaking were difficult. Eventually her fiancé, a medical student, read about myasthenia gravis and she was correctly diagnosed in 1927. 'There was at that time no known treatment and therefore many things to try.' She had gold injections, thyroid, suprarenal extract, lecithin, glycine and ephedrine. The last had a slight effect. 'Then in February 1935, came the day that I shall always remember. I was living alone with a nurse . . . It was one of my better days, and I was lying on the sofa after tea . . . My fiancé came in rather late saying that he had something new for me to try. My first thought was, "Oh bother! Another injection, and another false hope." I submitted to the injection with complete indifference, and within a few minutes began to feel strange . . . when I lifted my arms, exerting the effort to which I had become accustomed, they shot into the air . . . every movement I attempted was grotesquely magnified until I learnt to make less effort . . . it was strange, wonderful, and at first very frightening . . . we danced twice round the carpet. That was my first meeting with neostigmine, and we have never since been separated.'

Rheumatoid arthritis:

'When I was 52, my fingers, wrists, and feet, and especially my toes, became very painful and swollen with arthritis. I could no longer sew or knit, or do ordinary housework; writing was painful, and I could not walk in comfort . . . The worst of arthritis is that as one joint improves another

M.Y.T. — B

is liable to become painful . . . the back of my head, my neck, jaw, and right shoulder, and my back below the shoulder-blade, began to give trouble especially at night. If I sat up in bed the pain was bearable, but if I slipped down during sleep I woke with an agonizing headache. The pain was unbearable if I lay on my side; so I found it more comfortable to spend the night sitting in an armchair . . . Writing became more difficult, and it was almost impossible to dress myself or cut up my food. Yet I felt I must do these things for myself as far as possible, or I would become useless.

'The mornings were my worst times, and I felt quite helpless on waking: . . . I have not been so intimate with arthritis for eight years without learning a few ways of managing it . . . Aspirin is my great ally, the best of all the drugs I have tried . . . I don't feel life would be bearable without this.'

Severe pain afflicts many thousands of people daily both in and out of hospital. Morphine, an ingredient of crude opium from the opium poppy, remains a principal remedy despite the advances of synthetic chemistry. It is purified and provided in sterile ampoules for injection. Without morphine and its synthetic allies, surgery would be confined to the gravest conditions for the patient could not bear the post-operative pain.

A doctor victim of *coronary thrombosis* writes:

'It was on a grey, dull, Sunday morning at 7.30 that it hit me; and hitting is not a bad description. I was 48, and in the last twenty years I had not had a single day in bed. Two months before, I had woken early in the morning with pain in the front of the chest . . . It lasted about ten minutes. This was something new to me and I consulted one of my local colleagues, a very good doctor. The result of an exhaustive overhaul was completely negative: "Can't find a thing the matter, old boy; probably some indigestion; cut down the smoking", and so on.

'To revert to that Sunday morning: the pain was severe, very, centring on the middle of the chest . . . It was a gnawing, screwing pain – as if someone was applying a vice . . . and it gradually got worse. I was alone . . . I got out of bed and walked up and down, but it was no use; any drugs were downstairs and I could not, or would not, go and get them. "Besides," I thought, "I can do nothing"; and as I had never taken anything except aspirin and alkalis [for indigestion] in my life and was going to die in any case, why bother? But I wished it would hurry up; . . . I hugged the side of the bed, and then I must have passed out, for the next thing I remember was seeing my old factotum with the morning tea. She took one look and grabbed the telephone. My partner arrived and pushed some morphine into me – what a joy and relief! . . . Later, I read all the literature on coronary thrombosis I could lay my hands on . . . and was neither enlightened nor amused . . . and so I turned to P. G. Wodehouse.'

Asthma, a condition in which the bronchial tubes are contracted so that the flow of air in the lungs is obstructed may 'seem but a minor disability' when compared with many other diseases 'and indeed in a way it is. But not to the victim', writes a medical asthmatic.

'The importance of a disorder within one's own personal universe is measured by a different rule from that one applies to the illness of others. Asthma is certainly a major factor in my life, as it must be with most sufferers. But the numerous physicians with whom I have discussed my own case and those of my asthmatic patients have never seemed to appreciate the extent of the handicap. "You are all right between attacks?" they ask, and we usually reply inaccurately that we are. "Good," they say; "well, this will lessen the frequency and intensity of the attacks . . . And you know," they conclude happily, "no one ever died of asthma."

'I do not want to be unfair to my colleagues, and I know I must have treated patients much in this way. The reason is plain enough. Asthma is a condition in which successful therapy is extremely difficult, as can be seen from the great variety of treatments.' But 'adrenaline, of course [gives] relief' in acute attacks. In the 25 years since this was written substantial advances have been made in treatment of asthma by adrenocortical steroids which suppress the allergic inflammatory condition of the bronchi, by salbutamol (Ventolin) which dilates the bronchi like adrenaline but with less unwanted effect on the heart, and by sodium cromoglycate (Intal) which reduces the effect of allergic (antigen/antibody) reactions, which release bronchoconstrictor substances. In addition highly effective and convenient inhalers have been developed to deliver drugs directly to the bronchi.

Hay fever is an allergy to pollen.

'Those who have not experienced severe hay fever regard it as trivial, even a subject for jokes. But untreated it disrupts pleasure and even work for weeks on end.

'To picture the distress you must imagine your nose insufflated with pepper, or clamped with a clothes pin, or both. Clear fluid pours out and a dozen handkerchiefs a day may be soaked. Even if the pollen concentration is not high, so that symptoms are short of maximal, many things may trigger a sneezing fit: stooping, smoking, a single alcoholic drink, the scent of certain plants, a woman's perfume, dust, smoke, sleeplessness, sex. I was lucky in never having an asthmatic wheeze as well.

'In the nineteen thirties there was ephedrine (a feeble palliative, and an obstacle to sleep at night), adrenaline (impractical) and . . . desensitization. I was sent in my teens to an enthusiastic advocate of this and a fluent writer on hay fever. I must have given myself a course a year for over 25 years. Perhaps I owe my present relative freedom (or controllability) of grass hay fever to these injections, but there was no miracle. Once, when I was 21, and a combination of several of the factors I have mentioned gave me a terrible night, I walked over to the house of my doctor to show him that this method was not infallible. He was rather angry, muttered, "You can always control it with adrenaline" and got rid of me. It was a lesson, at any rate, that we none of us like to be confronted by our failures.'

Eventually in the late 1940s adrenocortical steroids became available as a result of brilliant chemical research and technology. The sufferer tried one; 'the result was miraculous . . . I have used it when necessary ever since . . . I now no longer dread the hay fever season.'

Diabetes mellitus: A standard medical text of 1907 states,

'Diabetes is in all cases a grave disease, and the subjects are regarded by all assurance companies as uninsurable lives: life seems to hang by a thread, a thread often cut by a very trifling accident.' Nowadays a young diabetic who requires daily injections of insulin because of failure of his own insulin production is accepted by most, if not all, life assurance companies with no or only a moderate financial penalty; he may have to pay the premium of a healthy person 5-10 years older.

Insulin was discovered in 1921 and first administered to man on 11 January 1922; it was then and is still derived from animals (pancreatic gland).

In the Preface to *The Diabetic Life*, a standard book for both patients and doctors written in 1925, the author, Dr R. D. Lawrence, himself a diabetic, wrote:

'Five years ago the "Diabetic Death" would have been a more suitable title for such a book as this. But now modern discoveries, particularly insulin, have completely changed the outlook. There is no reason why a diabetic should not ... lead a long and normal life[10] ... In conclusion, I would point out to diabetics and their friends that they owe their lives to medical research, and it ought to be their duty and pleasure to support it in further progress.'

It is estimated that there are 200 million diabetics in the world.

The young diabetic whose natural production of the essential hormone insulin has failed suffers from accumulation of toxic acid (ketone) substances in the body.

'The earlier symptoms are mainly digestive, nausea, lack of appetite, vomiting, colic and abdominal pain. When a diabetic who formerly had a healthy appetite suddenly loses it, the presence of a dangerous degree of ketosis must be suspected. Giddiness, irritability and restlessness are other symptoms, but an unnatural drowsiness is much more common. Great breathlessness apart from exertion is a more serious symptom,

---

[10] Unfortunately even careful management does not prevent some complications of diabetes: administration of insulin is thus not a complete answer.

the typical respiration being deep, heavy, and gasping (air hunger). It is caused by the stimulation of the respiratory centre in the brain by the acid bodies. If the patient be untreated, or even despite treatment in the pre-insulin days, he becomes partially and later totally unconscious and dies in a condition of profound coma and collapse. Insulin is able to recover most cases, and nothing is more dramatic in modern medicine than to watch the apparently dead come back to consciousness and life.'

However, diabetics will prefer not to be the subject of such edifying demonstrations and the correct use of insulin enables them to lead virtually normal active lives, in which the occurrence of coma is a rare accident, if indeed it ever occurs, rather than an expected complication.

R. D. Lawrence,[11] a pioneer in the management of diabetes, and especially in teaching the patient to manage his disease for himself tells how his illness began about 1920:[12]

'Many doctors, after they have developed a disease, take up the speciality in it. In the past, most superintendents of TB sanatoria were tuberculous themselves. But that was not so with me. I was studying for surgery when diabetes took me up. At that time I was house surgeon to the Ear, Nose and Throat Department . . . But before the sulpha drugs and the antibiotics, there were very many deaths in this department from mastoids and intracranial sepsis. It was my habit, and I think it was a good one myself, although it didn't pay me very well, to go to the post-mortem room at night and dissect the trouble that had gone wrong and find out why they had died, and to practise the operation on the other ear. Some people might think this gruesome. I had no time for thoughts of that sort. At any rate, chiselling away one night, I got a chip of bone in my eye. It went violently septic, and I had to be warded . . . Now for years, when going past [this ward] I've hated to look in at the door because it reminded me there was no good treatment for eye sepsis in those days, except by washing them out and

[11] R. D. Lawrence (1892-1968), physician, King's College Hospital, London.

[12] *King's College Hospital Gazette* (1961), *40*, 220. Transcript from a tape-recorded talk to the students' Historical Society.

that was a most painful process. Things got worse and worse. I had several operations – punctures for pus in the anterior chamber [of the eye, the space between cornea and lens].

'That brings me to the unusual happening. I don't know if they do it in every ward, but the night staff nurse used to teach the probationers how to test urines. They happened to take mine one night, and found it loaded with sugar – a great surprise to everybody. Next day the biochemist, Dr Harrison, did a blood sugar. It was three times the normal, so there was no doubt I had diabetes, which is probably why the eye sepsis got worse and worse and worse. You mentioned the Allen treatment, I got the Allen treatment all right. Starvation, absolute starvation, until you got sugar free. I believe I got sugar free in a week, but I was not interested in those days in the details of diabetes. Starvation got me fairly sugar free, and the eyes quickly got better. I've only got one eye now, but you can get along very well with one eye as long as it lasts. It's lasting very well, thank you . . .

'Well this was a great surprise to everybody as I had been looked upon as a fit sort of fellow. I played hockey and tennis for King's College Hospital, I believe I was captain of hockey, so I couldn't have looked very ill, and I certainly wasn't. I had no symptoms . . . There was one thing perhaps; whilst studying at night I used to fall asleep far too readily. But, of course, and I think you will all agree here, that is perfectly physiological when you are revising and studying such dull stuff as anatomy. You agree with that. That's not a symptom of diabetes. My God, it's too commonplace for that! It's a student's disease, isn't it? After that I stopped any idea of going in for surgery, and went into the lab., and learned a fair amount about it, and began to study medicine. But whenever I studied hard the tolerance [of the disease], which was fairly good for a bit, got worse and worse. When I began to read about diabetes and the Allen treatment and the great book of Joslin[13] . . . and when he said, in the 1919 edition, that by the Allen treatment of starving on a very low diet you might live three years with luck, and in the 1920 edition he said four years with luck, I found that was very depressing. It was quite obvious that when I worked

[13] E. P. Joslin (1869-1962), physician, Boston (USA), specialist in diabetes.

and my sugar got worse, the prognosis was extremely bad. I gave up all thoughts of working hard for exams and medical school life, and wanted a quiet, easy practice, where I could just live as long as I could.

'One thing I wouldn't do was to go home and die, with all the anxiety and horrid tension in one's own home. So I set about trying to get an easy life for myself. I was advised . . . that I should go to Florence, and be a general practitioner there . . . So off I set to Florence with a dictionary, a stethoscope, and *Gulliver's Travels* in Italian. That is the best way to learn a language – get a book you know fairly well in English, translated. I wanted to take the Bible, but it wasn't well translated into Italian, and so I thought *Gulliver's Travels* was very much better. I got on fairly well there and I was quite fortunate. I got a good consulting room in the main street, and began to get patients . . .

'I was pretty fit and well, and enjoying life and the art of Florence, until I got bronchitis. And then downhill as always happens; got full of sugar and acetone; lost weight; got so weak that I couldn't walk upstairs and I would fall down, and altogether things were getting pretty horrid. I would even fall asleep when interviewing a new patient. That tells you how bad I was with the acetone. A new patient in those days to me was a terrific event, and they were not plentiful. There were a lot of English residents there, and travelling English ate most unsuitable food and drank far too much Chianti, and so they needed my attention very frequently.

'So I was ready for anything. Dr Harrison, the biochemist, a great fellow, wrote to me and said there was something called "insulin" appearing with a good name in Canada – what about going there and getting it. I said no thank you; I've tried too many quackeries for diabetes; I'll wait and see. Then I got peripheral neuritis [inflammation of the nerves leaving the brain and spinal cord and supplying the muscles, etc.], and that wasn't good for doing medicine. And even my cigarettes, I couldn't get the matches out of the box. It really was pretty nasty. So when he cabled me and said "I've got insulin – it works – come back quick", I bundled into my car. I managed to afford a car. It was remarkable. I don't know how the bank manager gave me the money, but he did. There was an Italian garage man wanting to come with me to see his son who kept a restaurant in Soho. So we set off. A pretty tough journey it was. He funked Paris and I had to drive. When we got over the Channel to the "wrong" side [of the road], he wouldn't drive at all.

'I landed up at King's [College Hospital] all right one evening, and he got [me] a bed in Casualty of all places. There was nowhere else to go. Good enough. I had a good sleep. It was not a precoma business, but just exhaustion from travel. I didn't have insulin that night, because I was going to be a good guinea-pig and have my blood sugar done before insulin. Next morning (22 May 1923) at 9 o'clock I was along at the lab. as soon as it opened. The technician girl, Miss Taylor, found my blood sugar about 400 (normal 60-100 mg per 100 ml). Acetone and sugar couldn't have been more in the urine. Dr Harrison came at 10, went to the fridge, took out a bottle of insulin, and we discussed in our ignorance what the dose should be. It was all experimental, for I didn't know a thing about it; neither did he, for he had only treated about three people. So we decided to have 20 units – a nice round figure. He shoved it in, and I didn't feel it at all. I thought that this was nothing compared with all the things I'd had in the war [1914-18] – tetanus and anti-plague and anti-all kinds of stuff. They're horrid; insulin isn't, you hardly notice it. It is good stuff. At any rate I had that at 10 o'clock and my urine was tested every hour. I had a nice breakfast that day. I had bacon and eggs, and toast made on the bunsen. I hadn't eaten bread for months and months, and I did this without feeling guilty. It was really fine, and by 3 o'clock in the afternoon [my urine] was quite sugar free. That hadn't happened for many months. So we gave a cheer for Banting and Best.[14] But I didn't feel any different, neither better nor worse. However, at 4 p.m. I had a terrible shaky feeling and a terrible sweat and an awful hunger pain. That was my first experience of hypoglycaemia (blood sugar concentration below normal). However, having been sugar free, we remembered that Banting and Best had described an overdose of insulin in dogs. So I had some sugar and a biscuit or two and soon got quite

[14] The discoverers of insulin; one of the most famous and dramatic episodes of medical discovery: Sir Frederick G. Banting (1891-1941), Canadian (Toronto) surgeon and physiologist: Dr C. H. Best (1899-   ), physiologist (Toronto).

well, thank you. But next morning [my urine] was full of sugar again. With old soluble insulin it had to be given twice a day, and I still think it's the best treatment ever, though a bit of a nuisance as some people think. However, people who have been very ill and wasted and nearly dead would have had a hundred injections a day if it had made them feel as well as it did.

'Then I got a room somewhere nearby and really lived in the lab. and learned a good deal about even biochemistry. There was, of course, every week more insulin available and more diabetics put on it. So there was a great and growing crowd always in the lab. There was hardly any room for any general biochemistry. It was nothing but diabetics sitting about waiting to have blood tests, etc. An awful shambles. So something had to be done about it, and the first require-ment was for out-patient teaching. I must say the medical staff were very co-operative [he started a special diabetic clinic for which he had to raise money] but it wasn't so difficult to get as I expected. At that time there was a lot of money in London – London was a rich place and there were many rich diabetics who had been rescued from death by insulin treatment, and I had a good many of them as patients. One explained the necessity of this new treatment having new accommodation, and sent them a nice letter . . . and said you are very fortunate, you are one of the twenty men who are going to have the honour and pleasure of giving £500 [most of them became founder members of the Diabetic Association]. And they paid up very well, except Mr H. G. Wells.[15] I don't know if he was feeling a bit hard up, and in any case his diabetes wasn't bad enough to make him too sorry for himself, but he wrote a letter to *The Times* asking for money, and that did very well . . .

'At one time in early 1923 the insulin (standardization) was extremely bad. Some batches would be nearly twice as strong as others. Miller and I used to test new batches before, on ourselves. Thank goodness they soon got a good rabbit animal test,[16] so we did not have to function any more.'

In addition to the strictly humanitarian aspects of thera-

[15] H. G. Wells (1866-1946), novelist, philosopher, historian.

[16] The use of animals for testing drugs is discussed later; but we think such use is ethically justifiable.

peutics, there are *economic consequences* of sufficient magnitude to concern society. Healthy and happy people are productive of economic gain.

Peptic ulcer (duodenal 80%, gastric 20%) is an unpleasant condition. Sufferers are disagreeable to themselves, to their families and companions and they cannot work.

A sufferer writes:

'I was only 18 when I had my first attack of duodenal ulceration . . . the pain came with clock-like regularity three hours after meals . . . The next attack occurred twelve months later during a holiday . . . [it] had a serious consequence. I now became preoccupied with my health . . . apart from occasional pain, I was rarely free from abdominal consciousness . . . I experimented with diets. I resorted to patent medicines seduced by the advertisements . . . in early autumn I had my third and most severe attack. I must have been a pathetic object. Not yet 20 . . . [one] day immediately after lunch I was seized with a tearing agony throughout the whole abdomen. I struggled to the railway station; with board-like abdomen I could just gasp out a request for a ticket to my home . . . This was clearly a perforation . . . I need only summarize the ensuing forty-five years. There have been intervals of well-being with relapses of variable duration . . . it may be said that one's enjoyment of life is reduced by an ulcer to a greater extent than by some of the more serious disabilities . . . as George Meredith[17] says . . . one is not altogether fit for the battle of life who is engaged in a perpetual contention with his dinner.'

In addition to the chronic misery caused by duodenal ulcer, 6,000 to 10,000 lives are lost annually from the disease in the USA (population 217 million) mainly from bleeding or perforation; many cases require unpleasant major surgery with a fatality rate of up to 3% and a recurrence rate also about 3%.

Recent estimates suggest that 4 million people in the USA suffer from peptic ulcer and that medical care for these people plus the earnings they lost because of illness and death cost $3,200 million in 1977, in which year 6,400 of the

[17] George Meredith (1828-1909), novelist and poet.

sufferers would die of the disease and 81,000 would be unable to work. It is evident that effective treatment, by any means, drug or non-drug, would be welcome on grounds both of benevolence and economics.

Sufferers from the disease have long known that neutralization of stomach acid with alkalis, e.g. sodium bicarbonate, relieves their symptoms, though it does not generally hasten healing; innumerable indigestion remedies are promoted to the public on an enormous scale. Stopping smoking and rest in bed have been shown to hasten healing; diet is irrelevant to healing though important to comfort.

Drug therapy has been disappointing, although liquorice derivatives have been shown to have some effect on healing. Recently the development of drugs that selectively block the substances in the body that stimulate the production of stomach acid, e.g. cimetidine (Tagamet) has given new hope that drugs may both relieve suffering and reduce the enormous economic losses due to peptic ulcer. These drugs (histamine H_2-receptor antagonists) are the outcome of a scientific programme carried out in industry during the last ten years. It will be some years before the full implications of these new substances are known. We must wait and see; but there are grounds for optimism.

In this chapter we have tried to show the enormous and undoubted benefits that mankind obtains from drugs or medicines by means of a few examples. We have also touched on some important areas in which the use of drugs is controversial.

SOURCES

The accounts of disease in this chapter are taken from the following sources and we gratefully acknowledge permission to quote them.

'Disabilities and how to live with them': *Lancet*, 1952.

Sick Doctors: ed. R. Greene: Heinemann, 1971.

The Principles and Practice of Medicine: W. Osler, revised T. McCrae: Appleton, 1935.

The Diabetic Life: R. D. Lawrence: Churchill, 1925.

A System of Medicine: ed. T. C. Allbutt and H. D. Rolleston: Macmillan, 1907.

3. Assessing the risks

Risks should not be considered without reference to benefits any more than benefits should be considered without reference to risks.

'Risks are among the facts of life. In whatever we do and in whatever we refrain from doing, we are accepting risk. Some risks are obvious, some are unsuspected and some we conceal from ourselves. But risks are universally accepted, whether willingly or unwillingly, whether consciously or not.'[1]

There are two broad categories of risk:
First are those that we accept by deliberate choice, even if we do not exactly know their magnitude, or we know but wish they were smaller, or, especially where the risk is remote though the consequences may be grave, we do not even think about the matter. Such risks include transport, or sports, both of which are subject to physical laws such as gravity and momentum; or surgery to rectify disorder that could either be tolerated or treated in other ways, e.g. hernia or cosmetic surgery.
Second are those risks that are imposed on us in the sense that they cannot be significantly altered by individual action. Risks such as those of food additives (preservatives, colouring), air pollution, and some environmental radioactivity are imposed by man. But there are also risks imposed by nature, e.g. skin cancer due to excess ultraviolet radiation in sunny climes as well as some radioactivity.
The motives for accepting risk are various and numerous and include the general attitude of individuals to life, to work and to pleasure. There are those who enthusiastically engage in or support caving or mountaineering or hang-

[1] Pochin, E. E. (1975), 'The acceptance of risk', *British Medical Bulletin, 31,* 184.

gliding and there are those who urge that these risks are unacceptable and, not content with themselves abstaining from those recreations, campaign to have them stopped or controlled.

That unnecessary risks should be avoided, seems an obvious truth but there is great disagreement on what risks are truly unnecessary and, on looking closely at the matter, it is plain that many people habitually take risks in their daily life that it would be a misuse of words to describe as necessary. This is not a problem that will be resolved simply or by further study, for there are genuine differences of opinion on absolute evaluation of risk, and differences between individuals on the evaluation of risk in relation to benefit for themselves.

It is also the case that some risks, though known to exist are, in practice, ignored except by conforming to ordinary prudent conduct, e.g. the employment of competent electricians and gas fitters in the home, looking before crossing the road, not accepting a lift in a friend's car if he is drunk. In the case of public transport the acceptance of monopoly is not generally felt to pose serious safety issues since the risks are so remote in even a relatively inefficient organization. In the case of air travel in the UK there are about two fatalities per million flights, and in the USA and Australia one fatality per million flights; the worldwide figure is 3-4 fatalities per million flights. There can be few passengers who seek out the figures for individual airlines and take them into account before making a booking. The reason for this is that the risks involved in flying by any reasonably reputable airline are so small as to be ignored by ordinary people, i.e. the risks are negligible in the sense that they do not influence behaviour. Also, it only needs an airline to have one or two big plane crashes, unlikely to be repeated, to alter its safety ranking.

In general it has been suggested that, in medical cases, concern ceases when risks fall below about 1 in 100,000 so that then the procedure becomes regarded as 'safe'[2]. In such cases, when disaster occurs, it can indeed be difficult for the individual to accept that he 'deliberately' took a risk; he feels 'it should not have happened to him' and in his distress

[2] Ash, P. J. N. et al *Community Health*, 1976, 8, 29.

he may seek to lay blame on others in cases where there is no fault or negligence, only misfortune.

The benefits of chemicals used to colour food verge on or even attain negligibility, yet our society, on somewhat weak evidence, considers the risks are also negligible since it permits their use. A widely used food colourant, tartrazine, is known to cause an allergy (asthma) in man. It is unnecessary, but it continues to be used. The benefits of oral contraceptives and of penicillin are undoubted and the risks are equally undoubted and have been measured, and their use continues and expands because the benefits outweigh the risks. In no countries are the risks of heroin dependence (addiction) acceptable, but in all countries the risks of tobacco are acceptable or, at least, accepted. Deaths from uncontrolled tobacco dependence far exceed those of therapeutic agents and those of road transport.

The risks of drugs have become a major topic of concern over the last twenty years, and this concern, often amounting to alarm, has accelerated since the thalidomide disaster of 1960-1 which provided an exceptionally dramatic demonstration of the worst that drugs can do.

There is general agreement that drugs prescribed for the treatment of disease are themselves the cause of a serious amount of disease (adverse reactions). Classification is fundamental to all science, for without it we are intellectually lost, unable to think rationally about a subject, yet classification is peculiarly difficult in the field of adverse drug reactions. This is not surprising when we consider the enormous variety of drugs in use for diseases of even greater variety, and the fact that adverse reactions occur not only as a result of the intrinsic chemical properties of the drug itself and the amount given, but other factors involving the patient, the disease and the environment determine whether an adverse effect may occur in any one patient on any one occasion.

What follows is an attempt to provide *a framework for thinking about adverse reactions.*

1. NON-DRUG FACTORS

(a) *Factors intrinsic to the patient*

(i) *Age.* In the old, capacity to metabolize drugs (to alter them chemically, chiefly in the liver) declines and it has been shown, for example, that there is delayed metabolism of many drugs. Kidney function also declines with age and elimination of drugs from the body by this route is less efficient. Both these factors lead to increased concentrations of drugs in blood and other tissues and to increased incidence of adverse reactions.

It is uncertain how far increased sensitivity of organs may also contribute to increased responses to drugs seen in the old. In some cases, for example, hypnotics and sedatives and drugs for high blood pressure, the capacity to compensate for excess effect (oversedation, low blood pressure) may be limited and so give a false impression of increased sensitivity of the organs on which the drugs are intended to act.

In the first month of normal life the capacity for both kidney elimination and liver metabolism is relatively undeveloped, and this is even more marked in premature babies. Elimination of many drugs is therefore reduced. The failure of the newborn both to metabolize chloramphenicol (an antibiotic) in the liver and to excrete it via the kidney is particularly notorious and has resulted in death from toxicity to the heart and circulation, following well-intentioned attempts to prevent bacterial infections.

(ii) *Sex.* Whilst differences between human sexes in the rate of drug metabolism have been shown, they are probably not of importance in the occurrence of adverse reactions. Marked sex differences in toxicity at high doses have been shown in animals but no conclusive instances have, as far as we are aware, been shown in man.

(iii) *Genetics, including racial differences.* The basis for the familiar range of individual variation, the continuous variation of the normal distribution curve (single humped, like a dromedary camel), is genetic, and results from many gene inheritance (multifactorial), e.g. if a standard dose of a hypnotic is given to 100 people, a few will experience no effect, a few will sleep too long with severe hangover but the majority will experience graded effects between the extremes and will sleep moderately; the effects of alcohol in standard dose are well known to be subject to similar individual variation.

Where drugs are given in arbitrary fixed dosage the clinician is sometimes surprised at the occurrence of unexpectedly intense effects and asks whether the patient is 'hypersensitive' to the drug, when the effect is accounted for by the patient being at the lower tail of the normal distribution curve.

The most dramatic differences result from single gene (monofactorial) inheritance and give rise to striking differences that do not lie on a normal distribution curve.

Adverse reactions due to monofactorial (single gene) inheritance may differ in amount as in the bimodal (double humped, like a Bactrian camel) distribution curve of slow and fast metabolizers (acetylators) of isoniazid (a useful antituberculosis drug) or there may be a qualitative difference, as in the haemolytic (dissolution of red blood cell) reaction to primaquine (an antimalarial) due to a deficiency of the enzyme glucose – 6-phosphate dehydrogenase in the red blood cells; the effect is either present or absent, it is not graded, as on a normal distribution or a bimodal curve.

Plainly, genetic differences are likely to be recognizable between races. In the case of multifactorial (many gene) inheritance individual variations within racial groups are of size rather than of kind and it requires large studies to detect any differences between groups, and we do not know of medically important examples.

But, in the case of monofactorial inheritance, there are well-documented examples of racial differences that can be measured precisely. The haemolytic reaction to primaquine occurs in 5-10% of Negro males and is absent in North European Caucasians. Slow metabolism (acetylation) of isoniazid, with consequent higher blood levels and greater risk of adverse reactions, occurs in 5% of Eskimos, 15% of Chinese, 45% of Europeans and 60% of Asian Indians.

Failure to metabolize (hydrolyse) succinylcholine (used to relax the muscles and so render both anaesthesia and surgery easier) with resultant prolonged paralysis (hours instead of minutes) due to the presence of an atypical enzyme in the blood (plasma cholinesterase) occurs in about 2% of Europeans and is absent in the Japanese.

The occurrence of allergic reactions to drugs, when the drug or a breakdown product (metabolite), sometimes in combination with a body protein, forms an antigen (substance that stimulates production of antibodies), is probably also genetically determined.

In the course of introduction of new drugs that have undergone initial testing in a relatively uniform (homogeneous) population, it cannot be assumed that the dosage schedules and predicted adverse reactions that are defined in the country of origin will be the same all over the world.

(iv) *Disease*. The list of drugs the actions of which are modified by disease is extensive.

Adverse reactions are, as expected, more common in disease of the principal organs of chemical alteration of drugs (metabolism) and of elimination (excretion), the liver and the kidneys, and to give detailed examples would be superfluous; such disease constitutes a general hazard affecting a substantial proportion of drug therapy in those affected.

But disease of other organs is important; for example, the risks of opiates and sedative drugs in patients with malfunctioning respiratory centre (area of the brain controlling breathing) (advanced chronic lung disease, severe asthma), the precipitation of asthma by drugs used for angina pectoris (β-adrenoceptor blocking drugs), the occurrence of skin rash with ampicillin (Penbritin) (a penicillin) in patients with glandular fever, and of disorders of cardiac rhythm with digoxin (a standard treatment for cardiac failure) after myocardial infarction (heart attack), are but a few.

(b) *Factors extrinsic to the patient*

(i) *The prescriber*. It is obvious that the choice of drug and the skill with which it is used will have an important bearing on the occurrence of adverse reactions. There can be no doubt that many avoidable, and so unnecessary, adverse reactions occur due to insufficient skill and knowledge; the amount of necessary knowledge to practise medicine adequately over the full range of conditions presented to general practitioners is beyond the capacity of any ordinary individual to assimilate.

(ii) *The environment.* Environmental factors significant in causing adverse reactions to drugs include simple failure to restrict drugs to the intended recipient, for example halothane (a general anaesthetic) in the air of surgical operating theatres causes miscarriages amongst pregnant female staff, penicillin in the air of hospitals or in the milk of cows treated for mastitis causes allergic reactions in hospital patients and staff and in milk drinkers.

Drug effects may also be modified, usually reduced, by substances that stimulate the liver capacity to metabolize drugs (enzyme induction), e.g. insecticide accumulation (DDT), alcohol and smoking.

Antimicrobials used in feeds of animals for human consumption have given rise to concern in relation to the spread of drug-resistant bacteria that may cause disease in man.

Nutrition has been shown in animals to be capable of markedly altering the occurrence of adverse reactions. The definition of its importance in man awaits further study, but it has already been shown that high and low carbohydrate and protein intake modifies human drug metabolism.

2. DRUG FACTORS

(a) *Factors intrinsic to the drug*

(i) *Side-effects.* These may be defined as effects that are an inevitable part of the pharmacological action of the drug at therapeutic doses, but which are undesired, for example drowsiness from phenobarbitone when used against epilepsy, vomiting with digoxin or morphine, respiratory depression from morphine, low plasma potassium concentration (causing muscle weakness) from thiazide diuretics (used to increase urine output in heart failure and in high blood pressure), failure of male ejaculation with some drugs used for high blood pressure and so on.

(ii) *Secondary effects.* These are indirect consequences of drug action, for example yeast (thrush) infection of the respiratory tract or bowel as a consequence of elimination of the normal bacterial flora in the course of antibiotic therapy.

(iii) *Toxicity.* Toxic effects are due to a direct action of the drug, often at high dose, and a damaging effect on tissue is implied, for example liver damage from paracetamol (analgesic) overdose or from anti-inflammatory drugs used for arthritis; damage to the auditory nerve from streptomycin or gentamicin (antibiotics). All drugs, for practical purposes, are toxic in overdose and overdose can be absolute or relative; in the latter case an ordinary dose may be administered but may be toxic due to an underlying abnormality in the patient, for example disease of the liver or kidney.

(b) *Choice of drug*

Inappropriate choice can obviously be a cause of adverse reactions. It is in the hands of the prescriber who has already been mentioned above.

(c) *Use of the drug*

The technique of use of a drug can be important. It also is in the hands of the prescriber; obviously, unskilled administration of drugs where the concentration that produces the desired (therapeutic) effect is close to that which produces adverse effects (general anaesthetics, anticancer drugs) is more hazardous than unskilled administration of penicillin (for which the toxic dose is many times the therapeutic dose).

Drug regulatory authorities that collect and evaluate adverse reactions reported spontaneously by doctors seldom have information to allow them to determine whether an adverse reaction should be primarily attributed to the prescriber's choice or skill and so regarded as avoidable, rather than intrinsic to the drug and unavoidable.

(d) *Interactions between drugs*

Interactions can be classified into two main categories:

(i) *pharmacodynamic,* or interaction between the biological effects of the drugs at the target site, for example alcohol plus barbiturate hypnotic causing sleepiness or even coma.

(ii) *pharmacokinetic*, where one drug alters the plasma or tissue concentration of the other drug, the resultant effect on the subject being due to an interaction remote from the target site; for example the effect of an anticoagulant drug used for thrombosis may be seriously reduced by concurrent use of a barbiturate hypnotic because the latter stimulates liver enzymes which metabolize the anticoagulant more rapidly, thereby reducing its effect.

Within these two broad groups, interactions can conveniently be sub-classified according to the sites where they occur, thus:

Adverse drug interactions occur:

(i) *Outside the body:* for example antibiotics added to bottles of intravenous infusion solutions for slow continuous administration may become inactivated by the solution.

(ii) *At the site of entry into the body:* for example the absorption of tetracycline (an antibiotic) from the gut is prevented by calcium in milk and in gastric antacids; inhibition of the protective enzyme monoamine oxidase in the gut wall by some drugs used for mental depression leads to excessive absorption of some drugs or of substances naturally formed in cheese (tyramine), which can cause severe and even fatal high blood pressure.

(iii) *Inside the body,* after absorption: (a) *at transit and storage sites:* drugs are carried in the blood partly free and available to bind to active receptors, and partly loosely bound to blood plasma proteins and inactive; competition between two drugs for the binding sites on plasma protein can lead to fluctuations in amount of free drug available for action and so cause excessive effects of one of the drugs.

(b) *at site of action or nearby:* for example, some antidepressant drugs and appetite suppressants (for obesity) can reverse the effect of some blood pressure lowering drugs.

(c) *by interference with metabolism:* for example liver enzyme induction (see above) by barbiturates can cause failure of the low-oestrogen dosage contraceptive pill by increasing its metabolism.

(d) *at site of exit from the body:* for example changes in elimination of drugs by the kidney as a result of changing the pH (acidity/alkalinity) of the urine.

Some more detailed examples of what drugs can do will now be given to illustrate the range and complexity of the problems posed.

The chief adverse effects of drugs can be considered under three heads: death, permanent disability, and recoverable illness.

1. DEATH

Where a patient is seriously ill and likely to die risk-taking in therapeutics is plainly acceptable provided, of course, that the decisions are competent and are taken with appropriate patient or family participation.

But there is a definite mortality from familiar drugs used in a standard way, for conditions that may require drug therapy to relieve suffering or merely inconvenience, rather than to preserve life.

For example, *aspirin* is regarded as a safe and useful drug, and is taken in enormous quantities, but it can have effects at therapeutic doses, which though uncommon, result in a substantial amount of serious and even fatal illness.

In the UK (population 57 million) about 4.5 million people take aspirin at least once a week and about half a million take more than five aspirin tablets per day. It has been estimated that there are about 7,000 hospital admissions per annum due to acute bleeding from the gastrointestinal tract precipitated by aspirin, and some of these die. Evidence of causation is not unequivocal and it seems likely that an additional factor, e.g. alcohol, which increases the damaging effect of aspirin on the stomach, often plays a part.

Aspirin also causes minor loss of blood from the stomach in most people who take more than a few tablets and it has been calculated that in the UK the annual blood loss is about 90,000 litres (20,000 UK gallons, enough to fill a domestic swimming pool). Such minor blood loss, which over long periods can cause anaemia, may be detected by injecting into the circulation radioactive red blood cells. The appearance of radioactivity in the faeces provides a measure of bleeding into the gastrointestinal tract.

Aspirin, in ordinary doses, also occasionally causes other ill-effects, including asthma. But nowhere is it seriously advanced that aspirin is such a dangerous drug that it should be available only on a doctor's prescription and used only for serious conditions, e.g. rheumatoid arthritis. It remains a familiar and useful household remedy for pain, and rightly so.

It is worth looking more closely at what is known about this adverse effect of aspirin for it not only gives understanding of how drugs may produce adverse effects but also of how these may be mitigated by ingenuity.

About 1 in 15 of the population cannot take aspirin without risking gastric symptoms (heartburn, vomiting). Though some of this can be due to an action on the brain after absorption into the blood, most of it is due to a local effect on the stomach.

If an ordinary aspirin tablet is put on the lining of the mouth (mucosa) between cheek and lower jaw and allowed to remain there, after 30-45 minutes the mucosa begins to turn white, opaque, and to feel abnormal and a thin slough (area of dead tissue) that readily peels away may be formed. In the stomach, observed directly through a flexible optical instrument (gastroscope) passed down through the mouth and throat, the lining of the stomach (mucosa) shows congested, haemorrhagic areas where aspirin particles are lodged and the patient may or may not feel 'indigestion'. Even when aspirin is taken dissolved in solution (soluble aspirin tablets), as it should be, it causes increased shedding of the mucosal cells of the stomach lining (so do alcohol and mustard) and alters the quality of gastric mucus (the protective lubricant composed of long-chain molecules that slide over each other – saliva contains a lot, and the normal feel of the tongue sliding comfortably around the inside of the mouth is due to mucus).

When a tablet is swallowed it should rapidly disintegrate. Try dropping a (non-proprietary) tablet of (a) ordinary aspirin and (b) soluble aspirin into separate glasses of warm water and see what happens. The solubility of a drug determines how easily it is absorbed into the blood. Just as some stains can be removed from our clothes with water but others, fats and oils for example, require 'dry' cleaning, so some drugs are very soluble in water and others are more soluble in fat. Fat-soluble drugs are absorbed easily from the gut and water-soluble drugs less easily; wholly insoluble substances, like sand, are not absorbed at all. Fat-soluble drugs are absorbed easily because the cell walls of the gut, which the drug molecules have to pass through (by diffusion) are largely made up of fatty substances (lipoprotein).

Aspirin is interesting because it exists in two forms depending on the acidity of the solution it is dissolved in. In an acid environment such as the stomach aspirin is a fat-soluble substance (unionized) and so it readily diffuses into the cells lining the stomach. However, inside these cells the environment is now slightly alkaline. The aspirin molecule, being a weak acid, loses a positive electric charge (proton or hydrogen ion) in an alkaline solution, and so becomes negatively charged (ionized). These ions are water-soluble rather than fat-soluble and aspirin tends to accumulate in the cells lining the stomach because the water-soluble molecules cannot escape (by diffusion) as easily as the original fat-soluble molecules entered. This may explain why aspirin is harmful to the stomach. Damage to the cells may be directly due to the drug or to its facilitating cell damage by the hydrogen ions of gastric acid (hydrochloride acid). Gastric damage is enhanced by alcohol.

From the above it is evident that accumulation of aspirin in stomach cells may be reduced if conditions can be altered so that the drug is ionized during its stay in the stomach. This can be achieved by giving an alkali (e.g. sodium bicarbonate) to neutralize gastric acid at the same time as the aspirin is taken. There is evidence that such 'buffered' aspirin is less harmful to the stomach. The best-known of such preparations is Alka-Seltzer which consists of solid aspirin, citric acid and sodium bicarbonate. This becomes, when placed in water, a solution of sodium acetylsalicylate, sodium citrate and sodium bicarbonate. The sodium bicarbonate provides the necessary substantial (though transient) neutralization of gastric acid. Official soluble aspirin tablets do not contain enough alkali to reduce gastric acidity usefully.

Numerous other drugs can, even when properly prescribed, occasionally kill a patient unpredictably, e.g. penicillin, oral contraceptives, and the antirheumatic phenylbutazone (Butazolidin).

Penicillin kills by an immunological mechanism in a patient who has had the drug before and who has become sensitized to it, i.e. has developed antibodies so that when a subsequent dose is given the penicillin (antigen) combines with the existing antibodies. This combination results in damage to body cells which release biologically active molecules (amines, kinins) which can cause collapse and death by actions chiefly on the small blood vessels and the bronchial muscle (anaphylactic shock). It is to avoid this that doctors enquire of patients whether they have ever reacted unfavourably to penicillin, before prescribing it. But such a precaution, though prudent, is not sufficiently reliable to forestall all accidents.

The most effective *oral contraceptives* (containing two female hormones, oestrogen as well as progestogen) occasionally kill by causing the blood to clot (thrombosis) in vital arteries (heart wall, brain), or to clot in non-vital veins in, for example, the leg, whence the clot may break free and be carried to and block a vital vessel of the heart or lungs (embolism). The occurrence of such events, which are more likely in women over 35 years and in smokers, can be minimized by ensuring that patients with a history of naturally-occurring thromboembolism are not given these preparations and by noting and acting on early warning signs of thrombosis, such as pain in the calf of the leg, or of embolism, such as pain in the chest, and by keeping the amount of the oestrogen component as low as possible without losing efficacy. But even with such precautions some misfortunes will continue to occur. Long-term use of this kind of contraceptive is also associated with an increased risk of tumours of the liver.

Phenylbutazone (Butazolidin or 'bute') is a drug that effectively reduces the inflammation and pain of injury and arthritis. It does this by inhibiting the tissue enzymes that synthesize substances (prostaglandins[3]) which mediate the pain and swelling of inflammation; thus phenylbutazone is a 'prostaglandin synthetase inhibitor', and so is aspirin.

Phenylbutazone, by what is probably an immunological and unpredictable mechanism, can, rarely, cause destruction of the whole range of blood-cell-forming bone marrow (aplastic anaemia) or else, selectively, the elements that form some

---

[3] So called because they were discovered in what was thought to be the secretion of the male prostate gland; they are now known to occur throughout the body and to have important roles in physiology and disease (pathology).

white blood cells (agranulocytosis) that play an important part in protecting the body against bacterial infections. In Sweden (population 8 million) over 5 years, phenylbutazone and related drugs caused 14 cases of aplastic anaemia of whom 7 died. A person who takes phenylbutazone is also risking bleeding from his gut (especially if he has had a peptic ulcer in the past).

In addition phenylbutazone, taken over long periods, is suspected of causing a slight increased risk of leukaemia (a malignant blood disease). The drug is widely used for serious and disabling rheumatoid arthritis where the risks may be thought well worth taking. It is also taken for purposes that some would consider comparatively trivial, as in the case of the Duke of Edinburgh who revealed[4] that he took it to suppress the pain of arthritis in his right wrist in order to prolong his polo-playing capacity.

We do not express an opinion on the justification or otherwise of taking this risk for that purpose. But we suspect that the risk of polo may well exceed the risk to life of the drug. Both are real and both are remote.

It is evident that many people implicitly, if not explicitly, hold a view of life that could be summed up as 'Life is there to be lived. A preoccupation with remote risks accompanying ordinary necessary or pleasurable activities, including the taking of drugs for well-defined indications, will mean that life becomes a process in which avoidance of death takes precedence over positive living. Such a life is unworthy and not worth having.' We would only add that, if, holding such views, a person has the misfortune to be the victim of the rare drug-induced fatality or disability, there should be no recrimination because the risk was deliberately taken, or the risk was regarded as negligible, being so remote.

There are two principal types of *diabetes mellitus*, that occurring in young people (juvenile-onset) and that occurring in older people (maturity-onset). The juvenile-onset diabetes is due to lack of natural insulin production in the pancreas and is treated by replacement therapy, i.e. administration of insulin by injection. In maturity-onset diabetes the patient's tissues have become resistant to his own insulin and it is

[4] *Sunday Times*, 27 June 1976.

commonly treated with synthetic drugs taken by mouth. These either stimulate the production of insulin in the pancreas or else act on the tissues, affecting the absorption of sugar from the gut and its utilization in the body.

Whilst there is no doubt that these drugs improve control of the diabetes over a short period, the long-term effects on health and longevity have remained in doubt. The principal reason for this is the difficulty and expense of conducting a reliable study on large numbers of patients over years.

In the USA the National Institutes of Health conducted such a study on more than 1,000 patients over 8 years at a cost of $7.7 million in grants, plus the unassessed, but enormous, cost in time of physicians, statisticians, administrators and patients.

The results of the study suggested that some drugs taken by mouth for maturity-onset diabetes might shorten patients' lives, chiefly by causing premature death from disease of the heart and circulation. In an editorial in the *Journal of the American Medical Association* one physician assessed this at thousands of unnecessary deaths each year in the USA alone if the conclusions of the study are correct.

But the conduct and conclusions of the trial have become a source of enormous controversy. 'The design of the . . . study and the data [reported in November 1970] were both attacked and defended by medical scientists and bio-statisticians of equal credibility and integrity. The cauldron of controversy has been seething ever since.' Other smaller studies do not confirm the results of this large study.

The present position is that we still do not *know* whether these widely used drugs carry increased hazards for patients (in general, or for a particular sub-group) and it will probably be years before we do know.

In the meantime both doctors and patients are in a dilemma. The editor of the same *Journal* writes that he will assess each patient carefully, and explain the situation to him; for example, the patient may be offered a choice between swallowing tablets and taking the risk of this (whatever it may be), or of having tiresome daily injections of insulin. The editor writes, 'This is a classic example of having the patient participate – as an educated partner – in a therapeutic decision that involves the quality of life. Of course, I will have a "fully informed consent" form signed and in the chart.'[5] In other words, the decision to take a drug may now be becoming as serious and personal a matter for the patient as having a surgical operation (for which consent forms signed by the patient have been a routine requirement for many years).

During 1963-6 the death rate in young people with *asthma* in the UK rose rapidly; a less marked rise occurred in Australia, West Europe, USA and Japan. Investigations suggest that the cause was related to the development of new and more efficient ways of delivering to the lungs bronchodilator drugs in the form of inhaled aerosols (metered aerosols); one of these drugs in particular also affected the heart, and was used in a relatively concentrated form. Following warnings in the medical press, and (in the UK) prohibition of sale of these preparations directly to the public, the death rate fell, though in younger patients in 1976 it still remained a little higher than it was before the epidemic.[6]

The exact cause has not been found and may never be certainly known. The management of asthma has been changing over the past ten years with the introduction of more selective bronchodilator drugs and it seems unlikely there will be a recurrence of this epidemic.

2. PERMANENT DISABILITY

This may for some be as bad as or even worse than death, and drugs can do this too.

Partial or even complete *blindness* may be caused by drugs.

Chloroquine is an antimalarial drug that has benefited countless thousands of patients. Following a chance observation that arthritis improved when taking the drug, the use of chloroquine was formally explored in rheumatoid arthritis; it proved efficacious. But the doses needed for rheumatoid arthritis exceeded, over long periods, those customarily used to treat or to prevent malaria. Experience disclosed that prolonged use of chloroquine could damage both the cornea

[5] Moser, R. H. (1975), *Journal of the American Medical Association*, *231*, 1274.

[6] *Drugs and Therapeutics Bulletin*, 1976, *14*, 21.

(usually reversible) and the retina (usually irreversible) of the eye. Now, with the dose kept to a minimum and regular monitoring of the eye, this risk has been minimized. Chloroquine can also, rarely, cause serious muscle weakness.

In Japan, between 1956 and 1970 there occurred an epidemic of about 10,000 cases of subacute myelo-optic neuropathy (SMON). The name describes the disease (pathy); its onset was moderately rapid (subacute) and it affected the spinal cord (myelo), the optic nerve, and the peripheral nerves (neuro) to the limbs. Whilst some patients recovered, others have become permanently blind and paralysed.

The cause of this epidemic was not obvious. It might have been a virus, for example. Eventually, careful case studies implicated *clioquinol* (Entero-Vioform), used for bowel infections and diarrhoea, as *a* cause, if not *the* cause. Some uncertainty still prevails, but the balance of evidence points to the drug though perhaps not to the drug alone, but the drug plus some other factor (infection or environmental pollution).

The epidemic stopped when the Japanese Ministry of Health and Welfare withdrew permission for production and sale (September 1970).

But there remain puzzling features. Although the Japanese were using the drug in relatively high doses, some patients developed the disease at low doses, and the drug has been consumed in enormous quantities throughout the world for prevention and treatment of travellers' diarrhoea with little or no suspicion of toxicity. It was introduced into Germany, Italy, Japan and Switzerland in 1934, into the UK in 1947 and into the USA in 1954 but relatively few cases of SMON have been recognized outside Japan. Some apparent cases seem not to have taken the drug at all.

It therefore seems likely that, though the drug should be regarded as implicated, there is some other factor that contributed to this extraordinary episode with a drug that had even acquired, with enormous unsupervised use, a special reputation for innocuousness. A UK medical journal, *The Practitioner*, included in an answer to a query on travellers' diarrhoea (in 1964) that it 'appears to cause no adverse effects', and the *Prescribers' Journal* (published by the UK Department of Health, though written by independent authors) wrote (1964) of the drug that 'The public have bought it for many years with satisfaction and without harm'. Even in 1971 the *British Medical Journal* still felt able to entertain, even if a little remotely, the possibility that the Japanese cases were a complication of the disease for which the drug was given, rather than caused by the drug itself.

The controversial nature of the evidence is illustrated by the fact that regulatory authorities in different countries have responded variously, by continuing to allow the drug to remain available directly to the public, to be available on doctor's prescription only, or by total prohibition.

Whether other drugs of the same chemical group pose a hazard remains uncertain.

Kidney disease due to pain-relieving drugs (analgesic nephropathy) has been recognized after many decades of use of these drugs (the 'minor' analgesics or non-narcotic analgesics), e.g. phenacetin. These drugs are useful for the aches and pains of everyday life (headaches, 'rheumatic' pains, dysmenorrhoea). Phenacetin has been widely available on direct 'over the counter' sale to the public.

Mixtures of non-narcotic analgesics taken continuously over years can cause grave and often irreversible kidney damage. At first phenacetin alone was suspected, but other drugs, e.g. aspirin and caffeine, have been found to cause in healthy people shedding of cells from the kidney tubules into the urine. Drugs are greatly concentrated in that part of the kidney.

Analgesic nephropathy is most common in severe chronic rheumatism and in patients with personality disorder. The patients have been described as characteristically sallow, middle-aged women who smoke heavily, cannot sleep without sedatives, have recurrent ill-health and who have 'suffered dreadfully' from headaches for as long as they can remember. They have commonly had a broken marriage and may have attempted suicide. There are cases of mothers having introduced their daughters to analgesic-taking. The disease manifests itself as kidney symptoms, particularly passing water during the night and kidney pain; anaemia and high blood pressure are common.

Phenacetin abuse and toxicity. Although phenacetin was introduced in 1887, it was not until 1953 that suspicion was aroused that it might cause kidney damage. Certainty was not easily attained because, as well as the difficulties of interpreting associations discovered by retrospective enquiry, phenacetin is almost never used alone and it is hard to separate the effects of the several ingredients of mixtures. These mixtures have been widely abused, particularly on the European mainland, being taken for any trivial discomfort. The remarkable extent to which people can become dependent on them is shown by events in a Swedish town,[7] and these illustrate that drug abuse has emotional and social as well as pharmacological aspects.

During the influenza pandemic of 1918 a physician to a big factory in the town prescribed a powder containing phenacetin (0.5 g), phenazone (0.5 g) and caffeine (0.15 g). There was substantial mortality from the disease, but survivors thought they felt fitter and reinvigorated during convalescence if they took the powder. They continued to take it after recovery, in the expectation of becoming stronger and 'more nimble of finger', so that they would earn more in the factory.

Use of the powder, which could be got without prescription, spread through the town. Consumption increased and 'many families could not think of beginning the day without a powder'. It became almost as usual to offer a powder as a cigarette. When visiting friends in hospital, a powder 'was as welcome as flowers, fruit or chocolate, whatever the nature of the illness. Attractively wrapped packets of powder were often given as birthday presents.' Doctors regarded the habit 'as something of a joke'.[8]

The phenacetin consumption of the town was about 10 times as great as in a comparable (control) Swedish town. The deaths from kidney damage rose in the 'phenacetin town', but not in the control town, and in the decade 1952-61 there were more than three times as many.

An investigation was resisted by the factory workers and there was even an instance of organized burning of a questionnaire on powder-taking. It was eventually discovered that most of those who used the powders did so, not for pain, but to maintain a high working pace, from 'habit', or to counter fatigue.

There is no good reason to think phenacetin or phenazone

[7] Grimlund, K. (1963), *Acta Medica Scandinavia, 174*, supp. 405.
[8] *Ibid.*

effective for these, but each powder contained enough caffeine to give a noticeable effect (as in a cup of strong coffee), and as many as 10 to 12 powders a day were sometimes taken. The workers developed a considerable emotional dependence on the powders in the exact form in which they were accustomed to take them. Any slight change in the appearance of the powder rendered it, they thought, useless. Along with warnings of the danger of kidney damage, a clinic was set up to help people break their habit. At first those who went to it were subjected to 'persecution and derision' by their colleagues, but eventually the rising death rate brought home to the consumers the gravity of the situation, something that has not yet been achieved anywhere with cigarette smoking.

In 1961 phenacetin was withdrawn from sale to the public in Sweden and could only be obtained on prescription. The devotees of the powder changed to a phenazone, caffeine formula. When asked, they usually replied 'that it was quite useless, but that one had none the less to take a few now and then'. Sales of this powder, however, remained about the same as those of the original phenacetin-containing powder.

Sudden withdrawal demonstrated that there was no important physical dependence on the mixture, and the emotional dependence was probably a social, rather than a pharmacological phenomenon, though there is some evidence that phenacetin, as well as caffeine, can cause a psychic 'lift'.

Similar abuse has occurred amongst workers in the Swiss watch industry.

Most of the evidence that phenacetin causes kidney damage is circumstantial; attempts to reproduce the damage in animals have been only partially successful. The characteristic lesion is most commonly seen in patients with diabetes or overt recurrent urinary infection with or without urinary tract obstruction. Its occurrence in the absence of these factors is associated with a high incidence of heavy and prolonged phenacetin consumption.

Patients present with acute or chronic kidney failure and many improve when the analgesic mixture is withdrawn.

In addition, analgesic abusers may have a higher incidence of cancer of a part (pelvis) of the kidney. As with analgesic nephropathy, phenacetin is particularly suspected.

3

Paracetamol (derived from phenacetin) has now largely replaced phenacetin. It is not known with certainty whether paracetamol, used to excess, can cause kidney damage.

Pregnancy in women with epilepsy: In England and Wales 0.4% of all pregnant women have epilepsy and are under treatment with antiepileptic (anticonvulsant) drugs. The likelihood of congenital abnormalities in the fetus (chiefly cleft lip and palate, but also more serious anatomical abnormalities) is two to three times that occurring in fetuses of non-epileptic mothers. Death of the newborn (including still-births) are about twice as high in babies of epileptic mothers taking drugs as in healthy mothers.

The available evidence suggests that the standard anti-epileptic drugs are a principal cause of the fetal abnormalities and deaths, though the epilepsy itself may be a contributory factor. But the risks to the mother of reducing or stopping drug treatment of epilepsy greatly outweigh the risks of the drugs, and epileptic women who become pregnant are rightly advised to continue treatment.

An antiepileptic drug (sodium valproate) which was already widely used in France was introduced in the UK in 1974 although it was known to affect the fetus adversely in animal studies and so must be presumed to have a hazard to the human fetus. But the drug is effective in some patients who do not respond to the usual drugs. Risks can be minimized by selective prescribing, but they cannot be eliminated if the drug is used at all in women of child-bearing age. It will be extremely difficult to discover whether this drug alters the incidence of abnormality in fetuses of epileptic mothers.

Thalidomide will be discussed in the chapter on official control of drugs.

3. RECOVERABLE ILLNESS

Recoverable illness due to drugs is both common and of great variety. It ranges from nausea, drowsiness, vomiting and diarrhoea to life-endangering damage to vital organs. It can be dramatic in onset, e.g. sudden collapse from penicillin (anaphylactic shock) or insidious, e.g. gall stones (oral contraceptives) or gastric ulcer (antirheumatics).

Almost any natural disease can be mimicked by drugs.

M.Y.T. – C

The index of a standard work of reference[9] lists over a thousand adverse effects of drugs most of which, fortunately, are reversible.

SPECIAL PROBLEMS

There are three special areas in which a drug disaster might occur on a substantial scale. All result from interaction of the drug with the genetic material of the cell or its expression in cell division.

In all three areas there is particular concern because the effect may be delayed, difficult to recognize at an early stage and may be the same as natural disease and will therefore be difficult reliably to attribute to its cause.

1. *Teratogenesis* (teratos=monster: genesis=production) due to drugs taken during pregnancy.

This has already happened with thalidomide. The thalidomide disaster was dramatic, i.e. there was an epidemic of a rare, gross and consistent abnormality with the result that it was fairly soon realized that something new was happening, a cause was sought and comparatively easily found.

But lesser, though serious, abnormalities, especially if diverse in kind, could occur on a much larger scale before it was recognized that anything new or unusual was happening.

Increasingly, national registers of birth defects are being kept so that changes in incidence of abnormalities may be detected at an early stage. But these depend on easy recognition of the abnormality at or near birth. A drug, or other environmental factor, e.g. virus, could cause a drop in intelligence without this being noticed by any existing monitoring system.

For detection to be at all easy, positive suspicion must be aroused as in the case of thalidomide (dramatic abnormality), or of smoking (general suspicion) by mothers during pregnancy. Investigations suggest that smoking mothers have more still births and smaller babies, perhaps of slower development and lower intelligence. Another drug could be having effects of this kind in the community and remain unsuspected for

[9] *Meyler's Side-Effects of Drugs*, Vol. VIII, ed. M. N. G. Dukes, Excerpta Medica, Amsterdam, 1975.

a long time; indeed, unless its use was extremely common in women of reproductive capacity, an effect might well never be detected.

Extensive testing of new drugs in pregnant animals has been mandatory since the thalidomide disaster. At first, administration of the drug in early pregnancy in two animal species was thought sufficient. But now animal tests include administration before mating to detect effects on fertility of both sexes, administration throughout pregnancy, monitoring the birth and the development of the young animals through to maturity and testing their reproductive performance. How far such tests, especially when they give positive results only at the highest dose, provide genuine protection for man still remains uncertain. But as a consequence of thalidomide no new drug now reaches the market without such testing.

2. *Mutagenesis.* Drugs may cause abnormalities of genetic material (genes, chromosomes) of cells so that a permanent change in the hereditary constitution (mutation) occurs.

When a mutation occurs in reproductive cells (spermatozoa, ova) then a hereditary defect occurs. This defect may appear in the first-generation progeny of the individual, or it may be of a recessive kind that will only become evident if two individuals affected by the chemical mutagen mate. Thus the effect of a mutagenic drug might not appear for months or even years. The longer the interval the more difficult attribution of the true cause is likely to be.

Where a mutation occurs in somatic (non-reproductive) cells then these tissues, e.g. blood-forming bone marrow cells, may develop abnormal characteristics and become malignant (cancer); in the case of the bone marrow this is leukaemia. In this area of risk too, it can be difficult to establish a causal association with the drug which may have been taken and then stopped a long time previously; there is some hope of doing so where an effect is dramatic in frequency or in kind, but where there is merely a moderate increase in the incidence of a common condition then there is little prospect of detecting it and finding the cause.

Epidemiological rather than experimental laboratory techniques are required to determine what *is* happening in man rather than what *might* be happening. Medical record-linking schemes are being developed so that it will become possible, for example, to examine the drug history of all patients having a particular disease.

It is known that in appropriate experimental situations anticancer drugs, nitrite ion (used as a food preservative), caffeine (coffee) and ionizing radiation can be mutagenic, as also may be habitual tobacco smoking.

What is not known is how much hazard, if any, these pose to man in the actual conditions of real life. At present no systematic monitoring of populations for mutations is taking place, except insofar as birth defect and cancer registries may be recording effects of mutation.

In no country, at the time of writing, are routine tests for mutagenicity (in laboratory animals or isolated human cells) a mandatory requirement in the development of new drugs. That this is so is not evidence of lack of concern by either regulatory authorities or drug developers, it is because science is not sufficiently advanced to give a sufficient assurance of reliable prediction of what will happen in man.

This position is likely to change at any time. As soon as one country decides to require routine testing others are likely to follow. No body responsible for public safety cares to risk the accusation that it is being dilatory or unconcerned. Thus regulatory safety requirements grow and grow, often on only marginal scientific evidence.

3. *Carcinogenesis.* Malignant tumours (cancer) occur spontaneously and can also be induced by drugs and other chemicals, sometimes as a result of mutation.

The topic is extremely complex and controversial, but the possibility that drugs cause cancer in man is a major concern.

There are two important stages in carcinogenesis, initiation and promotion. Thus two substances may be necessary to cause cancer, an initiator and a promoter. But virtually any irritant substance seems to be carcinogenic in animals under the right experimental conditions. Glass, platinum foil, plastics, American dimes,[10] and strong glucose solutions have been found to be carcinogenic in animals.

Anticancer drugs are carcinogenic. They are often also teratogenic and mutagenic.

There is reason to believe that at least some cancers are the result of genetic mutations in the tissue cells causing a

[10] Moore, G. E. et al (1977), *Journal of the American Medical Association*, 238, 397.

hereditary change from normal organ cell type, e.g. liver, blood, to cancer cells.

Carcinogens may act directly on cells or secondarily through changes in the hormone balance of the body. Some cancers (e.g. prostate, breast) are hormone-dependent and male and female sex hormones are used in treatment, e.g. oestrogen for prostate cancer where the price of local comfort and longer life for the male patient may be the appearance of breasts of female size due to the treatment.

Animal tests to predict carcinogenicity for man are in wide use. They are required by regulatory agencies for certain groups of drugs which are under suspicion, e.g. oral contraceptives, for which 7-year administration to beagle dogs is becoming a usual test; alternatives are about 2 years to rats or 1 year to mice; that is, approximately life-long administration to the species concerned.

But for most drugs such studies are not, at present, mandatory. Debate on whether they should be is vigorous, continuing and inconclusive, indicating that their predictive value remains uncertain.

Since the appearance of cancer may be delayed until long after the drug has ceased to be used epidemiological methods will be required to detect the unexpected in man, i.e. cancer caused by a drug which is not under special suspicion. Where a drug *is* under suspicion then special investigations and careful monitoring of patients who have received it becomes practicable (cohort studies).

Recently there has been suspicion that a drug useful for high blood pressure (reserpine and other derivatives of the plant Rauwolfia serpentina) is associated with a higher than usual incidence of breast cancer. Reserpine has been found to be a 'promoter' in animal studies, i.e. if administered after an 'initiator' carcinogen it enhances the appearance of breast cancer. It also alters the hormone balance of the body in a way that is suspect as a cause of cancer, but which is similar to hormone changes occurring with some major tranquillizers and antidepressant drugs. Fears that reserpine causes cancer have receded following further studies. Plainly precipitate action by regulatory bodies at first suspicion can be unwise and unwillingness to accept any risk could lead to loss of useful drugs.

Chloroform, now little used as an anaesthetic, has been

used for over 100 years in medicines (it is also used in tooth-pastes) as a preservative and to mask unpleasant taste of other ingredients. As a result of tests in animals it is under suspicion for carcinogenicity and its use for inessential purposes is now increasingly prohibited.

It might be thought reasonable that a drug should be banned if it comes under the slightest suspicion. But slight suspicions are easy to arouse and hard to verify. Definitive investigations are enormously time-consuming and expensive. Precipitate action on only slight suspicion (especially that aroused by laboratory experiments in animals) is likely to do more harm than good in disrupting medical practice without corresponding benefit to patients. When a useful drug is under consideration to be banned then it is necessary to consider the alternatives that replace it and whether there is adequate knowledge of them; commonly there is not. This may at first sight seem a callous attitude but we believe it to be true to say that a blind 'safety at all costs' approach can in fact incur costs to patients in deprivation of benefits, costs that are excessive even in this important and emotionally charged area.

If it should occur that a new drug is found to be muta-genic or carcinogenic in man and that it had not been tested for these properties in animals before being introduced to man there can be little doubt that there will be a public outcry. Parallels will be drawn with thalidomide. The drug firm, and perhaps the national regulatory authority will be accused of negligence or incompetence.

It will be asserted that the possibility of a disaster was known (as it was), that laboratory tests for these properties existed (as they did) and that to fail to use them was plainly negligent (which is by no means necessarily the case).

The reason these tests are not yet mandatory routine for all drugs is that their predictive value is uncertain and that they are costly, though tests are, of course, required (regardless of cost) where there is positive reason to be suspicious, e.g. oral contraceptives. As is to be expected, the results are nearly always controversial. But at least new drugs in suspect areas should not give *worse* results in animals than similar drugs already in use.

The moment the predictive value for man is reasonably certain tests for carcinogenicity and mutagenicity will be generally imposed and indeed the drug industry will be only too ready to use them, however costly they may be. After all, it is the public, the patients, who pay in the end.

It is important (since it is in the public interest) that public fear does not push drug developers into doing, and regulatory bodies into demanding, massive testing programmes of dubious significance. On the other hand, public pressure for research into development of reliable predictive tests can only do good.

Until the science is more developed it should probably remain the case that carcinogenicity and mutagenicity testing is sometimes demanded and sometimes not.

In one well-known case a new drug (pronethalol) effective against serious heart disease (angina pectoris) caused cancer in one genetic strain of mouse but not in another; occurrences of this sort provide a nightmare situation for both drug developer and regulatory authority, especially if the drug will be used long term in man to control disease such as arthritis or epilepsy which do not seriously shorten life.

THE AMOUNT OF DRUG-INDUCED DISEASE IN THE COMMUNITY

When a patient takes a drug for illness and develops further symptoms or disease it is by no means always easy to determine whether the cause of the new trouble is the drug (which may be one of several) or natural disease.

A number of surveys have been done and estimates have been made, and it seems possible that as many as 3% of hospital admissions are due to adverse drug effects and that 10% or more of hospital in-patients suffer an adverse reaction during their stay. Unreliable though these figures may be, there is no doubt that a problem of considerable magnitude exists.

It has been pointed out that it is not enough to measure the rate of adverse reactions to drugs, their nature and their severity, though accurate data on these are obviously useful. It is necessary to take into account which effects are avoidable and which unavoidable. Also, different adverse effects can matter to a different degree to different people. In addition, prescribing patterns can vary greatly from one region of a country to another and there are substantial differences between countries.

Since there can be no hope of eliminating all adverse effects of drugs it is necessary to evaluate patterns of adverse reaction against each other. This can often mean that impossible comparisons are required. One drug may frequently cause minor ill-effects but be safe as far as life is concerned, though patients do not like it and may take it irregularly to their own detriment. Another drug may be pleasant to take so that patients take it consistently, with benefit, but it may rarely kill someone. Which is the treatment to be preferred?

Some patients, e.g. those with a past history of allergic disease or previous reactions to drugs, are up to four times more likely to have another drug reaction so that the incidence does not fall evenly on the population taking a drug.

The aim must be to discover the causes of adverse reactions, where these are unknown, and to use such knowledge to render what are at present unavoidable reactions avoidable.

Avoidable adverse effects will be reduced by more skilful prescribing and this means that doctors, amongst all the other claims on their time, must find time better to understand drugs, as well as understand their patients and their diseases.

Despite all this we are confident that drugs do far more good than harm.

The rest of this book is largely on the subject of reducing the risks of drugs.

RESPONSIBILITY FOR ADVERSE EFFECTS OF DRUGS

All civilized legal systems provide for compensation to be paid to a person injured as a result of using a product that is defective due to negligence (lack of proper care or attention) of its producer. But there is a growing opinion that compensation for personal injury should be automatic and not dependent on fault and proof of fault of the producer, i.e. 'liability irrespective of fault', 'no-fault liability' or 'strict liability'. After all, a victim needs assistance regardless of the cause of his disability and whether or not the producer deserves punishment. There is also the difficulty and expense of proof of fault or negligence which provides such extensive employment in the legal profession. Many countries are proposing legislation on the topic 'liability for defective products'. The UK Law Commission in 1977[11]

'set out the main considerations of policy that are relevant to the issue as to where the loss occasioned by a defective product should lie. These considerations comprise ideas of morality and justice as well as considerations relating to insurance, economics and administrative convenience.'

The major principle was expressed:

'Where a person suffers personal injury because of the defective state of a product, the loss should be borne by the person or persons who created the risk by putting the defective product into circulation for commercial[12] purposes, rather than by the person injured.'

It was represented to this body of lawyers that there were reasons for treating pharmaceuticals differently from other manufactured products, e.g. cars, can openers, etc. But it concluded

'that all the policy considerations in favour of imposing strict liability on producers apply with as much force to pharmaceuticals as they do to other products. The producer of defective pharmaceuticals creates the risk; he is the person best able to control the quality of the product; he is the person best able to insure against claims; and public expectation that drugs on the market will be safe is raised by advertising and by the promotional material with which the pharmaceutical industry supply the medical profession.'

In reaching this conclusion the Law Commission, in common with similar bodies in other countries, had taken adequate account of some, but not all, of the special problems posed by drugs.

If compensation is to be automatic on demonstration that

---

[11] *Report of The Law Commission and The Scottish Law Commission on Liability for Defective Products*: HMSO: London: 1977.

[12] It is to be hoped that this is not intended to exclude government responsibility where this is appropriate.

the product caused, or probably caused, injury then the cost of such compensation would become part of general production costs as is the case with some industrial diseases. Liability would only apply where there was a safety issue; other matters affecting products such as unsuitability for intended use and consequent economic loss would continue to be covered by laws of sale.

It is recognized that once liability no longer depends on fault, then innovators are faced with unpredictable and incalculable risks, especially in the case of drugs; and since the development of better drug therapy is in the public interest, it is also recognized that it will be necessary to limit compensation to levels that will not cause the innovators to withdraw from this already commercially risky, though sometimes highly profitable area.

The intention to apply such 'no-fault' or 'strict' liability to drugs may seem common-sense natural justice, but it raises special problems, for example:
1. Capacity to cause adverse effects is intrinsic to drugs.
2. Adverse effects (though often minor) are extremely common and severity extends over a continuous range.
3. Many adverse effects, including some of the most serious, are the same as naturally occurring diseases and it is often impossible in individual patients to distinguish between drug-induced disease and naturally occurring disease.

Drugs can be said to be 'defective products' by definition, that is, however well made, the capacity to cause damage cannot be eliminated because it is inherent. One or two refrigerators amongst the annual output of a factory may cause harm to the user, or a batch may have a design or manufacturing defect that is correctable once it has been discovered, but every aspirin is liable to cause harm to the user because it is an inherent property of aspirin to damage the lining of the stomach. Paracelsus[13] was right when he wrote: 'All things are poisons and there is nothing that is

[13] Aureolus Theophrastus Bombastus von Hohenheim, otherwise Paracelsus (1493-1541), Swiss physician, a forerunner of modern therapeutics. As Professor of Medicine in Basel he condemned medicine not based on experience and publicly burned the ancient works of Galen (129-199) and Avicenna (980-1037) which he considered at fault in this respect.

harmless; the dose alone determines that something is not a poison.'

Drugs may cause an increased incidence of a disease which already occurs spontaneously in the community. Currently available oral contraceptives increase the risk of coronary thrombosis and other clotting disease by their nature, but these diseases occur naturally amongst women, especially those who smoke. Women knowingly and willingly take the risk to reap the benefit. It is not practicable to define which patients would have got the disease anyway, if they had not taken the drug, and what account, if any, should be taken of smoking when deciding compensation.

Abnormalities in the newborn may be spontaneous or caused by drugs or other environmental factors, and except in the case of an epidemic of a rare abnormality such as that caused by thalidomide it is not possible to decide which abnormality is due to a drug and which is not. Thus it is hard to see how compensation would be allocated. But it is easy to predict the feeling of a mother who was told her baby with cleft palate or heart abnormality did not qualify for an award because it could not be proved that a drug she had taken in early pregnancy was the cause of the abnormality.

'Strict liability' laws applied to drug therapy generally would create two categories of disease, and it would be a matter of the greatest importance to the patient into which he or she was put, a category of disease that was compensatable because it was or could have been due to a drug, and a category, often identical in its manifestations, that did not attract compensation because it could not be assigned with reasonable certainty to a drug. And there would be no possibility of reliably assigning a high proportion of patients to one or to the other.

Also many adverse reactions are largely due to abnormalities in the patient, rather than to the drug, e.g. for most people penicillin is one of the safest drugs there is, but some, predisposed to allergy, occasionally get a rash, or rarely kidney disease, or even drop dead with anaphylactic shock. It could be said that it is the patient who is defective rather than the drug. Diseases of liver and kidneys particularly, render patients more likely to adverse drug effects.

Drugs are not offered as safe in the way that refrigerators are offered as safe; 'design defects' in refrigerators can be rectified once they are identified; this is not so for drugs, indeed the term 'design defect' is not applicable in the same way.

Drugs, the risks of which are well known, are often taken for convenience as well as from overriding need.

'It is acknowledged that some drugs are potentially dangerous and that many can have unpleasant side-effects and that it would not be appropriate to stigmatize them as "defective" on these grounds alone. A line must be drawn between the risks and effects which a person taking a drug may reasonably be expected to accept without complaint and those which are beyond what a person ought reasonably to expect. We believe that the standard of reasonable safety, discussed earlier, is an appropriate standard for determining whether the pharmaceutical product in question is "defective" for the purposes of imposing strict liability on the producer.'[14]

This standard of reasonable safety is expressed by the Law Commission in

'two propositions that we regard as fundamental, namely –
(a) a product should be regarded as defective if it does not comply with the standard of reasonable safety that a person is entitled to expect of it; and
(b) the standard of safety should be determined objectively having regard to all the circumstances in which the product has been put into circulation, including, in particular, any instructions or warnings that accompany the product when it is put into circulation, and the use or uses to which it would be reasonable for the product to be put in these circumstances.'

Application of these superficially extremely reasonable statements of general principles of reasonableness to the range of individual cases where drugs may have been taken from urgent necessity or merely for convenience is likely to prove impossibly contentious.

In the general practice of therapeutics, should the user accept the responsibility or should the manufacturer (pro-

[14] Law Commission Report: *ibid.*

vided that he has adequately informed the user, and provided he has supplied a pure product)? What is the position of the prescriber? Must he ensure that every known risk, however rare, is known to the patient? Should aspirin, sold over the counter to the public, carry a warning that at ordinary doses it can cause damage or even kill?

The list of questions is endless.

The laudable objective of the proposed law is to ensure that individuals who suffer should have their suffering compensated as far as possible. The question is how to achieve this without unintentionally causing suffering in other ways, e.g. distorting the proper use of drugs and stopping the development of new drugs in areas where they are needed.

We doubt whether a law that may be appropriate to ordinary manufactured products will also be appropriate, in the same terms, to drugs.

We suggest that the following would be reasonable:

1. With new drugs under trial and during any period of formal post-marketing surveillance the manufacturer has a responsibility for accidents that may occur, for the patients are taking risks, not only for themselves, but for the benefit of the manufacturer and, indeed, of the community.

2. With standard drugs, provided they are properly manufactured, promoted, prescribed and used by the patient, then adverse reactions should be regarded as part of the general medical condition of the patient; the patient will be cared for by the national health and insurance systems available for the sick.

3. Where healthy people are encouraged and persuaded to take medicines not only for their own good, but also for the good of others, as in immunization programmes for poliomyelitis, where there is a remote risk of paralysis not only of the recipient, but also of contacts of the recipient, then the victim should receive special compensation from the community (via government) beyond that of ordinary illness.

We doubt the wisdom of attempting to introduce 'strict liability' covering all, or all serious, adverse effects in all people (except in the case of new drugs under trial or surveillance). Creation of two categories of disease, one due to drugs for which money compensation is paid and the other 'natural' which will attract no special compensation will lead to injustice and will be unworkable. The difficulty of being sure in individual cases that disease is caused by a drug or drugs, and this is a very real difficulty, will be likely to lead to endless complaints, tribunals and litigation.

Surely it is best, where there is no negligence, that society should look after its casualties regardless of cause without trying the impossible, and therefore expensive, task of defining liability for disease between nature, the drug, the patient, the manufacturer and the prescriber, and compensating differentially. Similar disabilities need similar help, regardless of the cause.

That society should look to its casualties must mean government taking responsibility in this area, whether this responsibility is related directly to drugs or diffused as general social security against misfortune.

In general, government (i.e. politicians and civil servants) does not hesitate to take powers, as a duty in the public interest, of course; but it also sometimes shows a marked reluctance to accept liability for any unpleasant consequences of the exercise of those powers, though glad enough to claim and accept responsibility when things go favourably.

Where government has taken power to control medicines, to forbid their supply until it has satisfied itself that the evidence of efficacy, safety and quality is adequate, then the question must arise whether government has also undertaken at least some 'strict liability'.

Government exercises power, as it must and should, and power ordinarily entails acceptance of responsibility. The spectacle of those with power seeking to evade responsibility for the consequences of exercising it is unedifying, but familiar.

On the other hand it may seem unreasonable that politicians and civil servants, providing, as they should, a safety screen for the community, in the knowledge that it must be incompletely effective, should be held vicariously liable for accidents even though they have used the best advice available. But drug developers also conduct their activities knowing that their science is imperfect; the public too knows this; it accepts with alacrity the successes, but is prone to resent the inevitable failures.

It is also the case that only governments and the very

biggest industrial concerns have the resources to cope with a substantial drug accident; though collective insurance by industry is being undertaken in some countries.

Issues of responsibility for harm due to drugs where there is no fault still need to be resolved, and a sensible attitude of the public is essential, for it is natural for elected politicians to seek to give the public what it wants.

The experience with practolol (Eraldin) provides a model of what can happen with a new drug and will be discussed in some detail.

Practolol belongs to a group of drugs (β-adrenoceptor blockers) proved to be beneficial over many years in a variety of serious diseases, angina pectoris, high blood pressure and disorders of heart rhythm including those associated with coronary thrombosis. Since it lacked certain disadvantages of the earlier members of the group, it became widely prescribed, it saved lives.

Practolol was developed to the highest current scientific standards; it was marketed (1970) only after independent review by the UK drug regulatory body. All seemed to go well for about four years (though skin rashes were observed; an effect seen occasionally with an enormous number of drugs, household chemicals, clothing dyes, etc.) by which time there had accumulated about 200,000 patient years of experience with the drug, and then, writes the then Research Director of Imperial Chemical Industries Pharmaceuticals, 'came the bolt from the blue and we learnt that it could produce in a small proportion of patients a most bizarre syndrome, which could embrace the skin, eyes, inner ear, and the peritoneal cavity'.

The cause is likely to be an immunological process to which a small minority of patients are prone; 'with present knowledge we cannot say it will not happen again with another drug.'

That the drug caused this peculiar syndrome (characteristic group of symptoms and signs) was recognized by an alert ophthalmologist who ran a special clinic for external eye diseases. In 1974 he suddenly became aware that he was seeing patients complaining of dry eyes but with unusual features. Instead of the damage being on the front of the eye exposed by the open lids it was initially in the areas behind and protected by the lids. He noted that these patients were all taking practolol. Quite soon the syndrome was defined, as above. Some patients have become blind and some have required surgery for the peritoneal disorder and a few have died as a consequence.

The drug is now available (in UK) only for brief use by injection in emergency control of disorders of heart rhythm. ICI Pharmaceuticals acknowledges moral (though not legal) liability for the harm done and has paid compensation to affected patients.

Commenting on this the *Lancet*[15] wrote:

'At the last count, ICI had compensated 300 of the 1,000 individuals claiming to have been harmed by the beta blocker, practolol. This episode evokes memories of thalidomide, but there are important differences. Unlike thalidomide, practolol had been assessed by an official body – the Committee on Safety of Medicines – which had pronounced itself satisfied with the drug's experimental and early clinical toxicity record. Furthermore, the nature of the practolol reaction is not understood, and there seem no animal or in-vitro tests which could have predicted it. Do these changes in drug-control practice influence the responsibility of a pharmaceutical company to compensate patients who suffer adverse reactions? A small group discussed this question last year at the Royal College of Physicians and their deliberations have just been published. The Research Director of ICI stressed the unforeseen nature of the practolol reaction: he reckoned that, assuming that there was a species of laboratory animal suitable for its detection, clear demonstration of such an association might demand experiments on 50,000 to 100,000 animals. It was also evident that, although clinical-trial methodology has developed to a high degree, assisted by the growth of clinical pharmacology as a scientific discipline, and despite the early-warning systems now operating to detect adverse effects at an early stage in the life of a drug, drug reactions easily escape notice when not predictable from known pharmacological actions of a drug or when they do not fall into a recognized syndrome of such reactions.

'But it is the legal aspect of the practolol episode which is the most perplexing. A lawyer interpreted the present

15 *Lancet* (1977), *1*, 788.

position in law to be that, in guarding against risks, "a manufacturer of drugs must take such care as a reasonably careful and skilful drug manufacturer would take . . . In English law he will not be negligent if he has acted in accordance with a practice accepted as proper by a responsible body of his peers skilled in the particular skill in which his field of activity lies . . . If he has performed all the tests contemporary science has devised and nevertheless something then goes wrong, he will escape liability in this country". While this may well be a true statement of law, many people will feel that a company has a moral responsibility to compensate patients for harm sustained from a drug which they have persuasively encouraged doctors to prescribe (and sometimes even patients themselves to request) with attractive claims of safety. But one difficulty, in every case, is to prove a causal association – particularly if some parts of the drug reaction, as with the practolol syndrome, are not uncommon in the absence of drug ingestion. ICI's offer of compensation, before questions of litigation were formally raised, is an admirable gesture; but there might have been some advantage in allowing matters to proceed to the courts. Unfortunately the practolol affair is unlikely to be the last of its kind, and clarification of the law would have been useful.'

Understandably, it has been asked why doctors failed to recognize the effects of practolol, particularly on the eyes. The answer is that when a drug insidiously increases the incidence of common symptoms, in this case mild eye complaints, suspicion is unlikely to be aroused in the minds of doctors, each of whom is using the drug on comparatively few patients; it is liable to be delayed until more serious or unusual effects occur.

It is now appreciated that it is going to be necessary to survey many thousands of patients taking new drugs, carefully recording all adverse events, however slight or apparently irrelevant, if early recognition of potentially serious but uncommon effects is to be achieved. The conduct of such surveys presents many problems, including expense.

4. How drugs act

All living things can be seen struggling to achieve 'self' or identity. These assertions of 'self' are often expressed by secretion of chemicals which are repellent or poisonous to other forms of life. Man's experience of these poisonous effects of plants and animals, paradoxically, has often led to the development of new remedies for treating his own diseases.

William Withering,[1] who defined the use of digitalis (foxglove leaves) in heart disorders, wrote in 1787, 'Poisons in small doses are the best medicines; and useful medicines in too large doses are poisonous'; i.e. *drugs are useful poisons*.

Bacteria, the simplest of free-living organisms, produce some of the most lethal poisons known to man. For example botulinum and tetanus toxins are several million times more toxic than strychnine. However, the really interesting thing is that bacterial toxins can damage and kill in many different ways. For instance, botulinum toxin produces respiratory paralysis, tetanus toxin produces muscular spasm and convulsions, diphtheria toxin damages the heart and the toxins of staphylococci rupture red blood corpuscles. Much has been learned about the way drugs act from studying these toxins. Happily, bacteria and fungi often produce substances which are toxic to other micro-organisms but not to man and these, the so-called antibiotics, have been a therapeutic gold-mine. Not all of the thousands of known antibiotics are useful to man, but finding out how they interfere with living processes has told us a lot about the way biological machines work.

Bacteria and fungi are not the only source of poisons; jelly-fish, starfish, sting rays, spiders, scorpions and snakes are all venomous animals, i.e. they produce poisons. The human species has had to contend with all of these and much

---

[1] William Withering, MD, FRS (1741-99), physician.

more besides. Poisonous plants must have been a bane of
its early life and even today the injudicious and the ignorant
are doomed by plant poisons. Just like bacterial toxins, plant
poisons can produce an enormous variety of effects in man.
Early man didn't know about bacteria but he soon knew
his onions, his tea and his coffee as well as his deadly nightshade. He must have learned very early that certain plants
could not only harm him but give him useful poisons. There
is no doubt that folk medicine was not all hocus-pocus. The
virtues of the opium poppy, deadly nightshade, the purple
foxglove and ergot from fungus-infected rye, employed in
old herbal remedies, are now used in modern medicine as
their purified active ingredients – morphine, atropine, digi-
toxin and ergotamine.

For centuries, it was known that eating ergot, the name
for the reproductive bodies of a fungus infecting rye grains,
interfered with pregnancy and it was used for inducing
labour. Ergot could also constrict the small arteries and when
eaten, as bread made from infected rye, for any considerable
time, could produce severe gangrene of the limbs. The disease
became known as St Anthony's Fire, because the long
journey to the Saint's shrine at Padua (Italy) was often
associated with relief, no doubt because victims escaped from
the supply of infected grain. It took man till the seventeenth
century to learn to avoid making bread from infected rye
but by the end of the nineteenth century he was still fumbling
to exploit its value as a medicinal herb in obstetrics.

The young Henry Dale,[2] fresh from his training by the
great physiologists of the day at Cambridge, brought modern
pharmacological science to ergot at the beginning of this
century with extraordinary success. First (1906) he found
that an extract of ergot had sympatholytic actions, that is, the
ergot extract could annul the blood-pressure-raising effect
of adrenaline (epinephrine). In fact, it reversed the effects so
that adrenaline now caused a fall in blood pressure. Adrenaline, as every journalist knows, is produced in the body in

[2] Henry H. Dale (1875-1968): his revolutionary studies in
physiology and pharmacology were carried out in industrial
laboratories (Burroughs Wellcome Ltd) and in the laboratories
of the Medical Research Council (UK): his collaboration with
the medical chemist George Barger (1878-1939) was vital to
success.

response to stress and changes the activity of every organ in the way most suitable to meet the emergency. The heart is stimulated to beat faster and the bowel is inhibited into quiescence; the pupils are stimulated to dilate but the bladder is inhibited; the blood vessels to the skin are stimulated into contraction so that blood can be shunted towards the muscles in arms and legs where the blood vessels are inhibited and dilated; the subject is ready for fight or flight. Dale found that his ergot extract was a partial or selective antagonist to adrenaline; the excitatory actions were reduced but the inhibitory actions were untouched. Paul Ehrlich[3] had introduced the idea of selective toxicity ('magic bullet', learning to aim with chemicals) twenty years earlier to explain how his arsenicals would poison parasites without destroying the host, i.e. chemotherapy. But here was selective toxicity occurring between the tissues of a single animal and this, as we will see, is the heart of modern pharmacology.

Dale went on to look at the chemical nature of his ergot extract and ergotoxine was the name given to the 'pure' substance found in it. Ergotoxine is now known to be a mixture of three different but closely related substances, all derivatives of lysergic acid. Another simple derivative of this substance, lysergic acid diethylamide, is better known as LSD_{25}, famous for its ability to disturb the human consciousness and produce hallucinations. But the sympatholytic actions, mentioned above, were found not to be the basis of ergot's stimulant action on the uterus in obstetrics; Dale had to wait nearly thirty years to see the agent responsible for this effect, another related derivative of lysergic acid, ergometrine (ergonovine), to be isolated from ergot.

Although Dale didn't find ergometrine in his ergot extract he did find two other substances which led to a revolution in pharmacology. Unlike the ergot alkaloids which are complex chemicals, these new substances, histamine and acetylcholine, were very simple. Dale showed that histamine acted on tissues and organs throughout the body to produce a picture almost identical with anaphylactic shock – though it took nearly thirty years to prove that it was actually respon-

---

[3] Paul Ehrlich (1854-1915) developed the concept of 'aiming with chemicals', i.e. selective toxicity (chemotherapy) and realized it in practice: he worked in Frankfurt, Germany.

sible for this dangerous condition.

Anaphylactic shock occurs when a foreign protein is given to a sensitized person. We become sensitized to a protein when our first-line defences for keeping foreign substances out of our system fail; if it penetrates, the second line of defence operates, which is the manufacture of new proteins called antibodies. These antibodies are 'designed' to recognize and combine with the foreign protein and they are fixed to the outer surface of tissue cells which make and store histamine. Anaphylaxis occurs when a second invasion of the foreign protein is detected and bound by the antibody; this binding of antigen to antibody makes the defending cell release its stored histamine. The histamine, in turn, opens up millions of pores in the blood capillary walls to flood the area invaded by the foreign protein with plasma and blood cells to dilute, neutralize and ingest the foreign molecules.

Histamine has many other actions on tissues which seem to be designed to repel invaders, but as in every war there are innocent victims; in this case there is also stimulation of secretion in eyes and nose, contraction of the muscles in the bronchi narrowing the airways (asthma) and dilation of blood vessels, leading to low blood pressure and shock; the whole reaction can be unpleasant, dangerous or even lethal.[4]

Dale's work not only led to this understanding of the pathology of anaphylaxis but, many years later, it also led to the development of drugs which would block the actions of histamine on tissues in much the same way as he had shown that ergotoxine blocked some of the actions of adrenaline. The antihistamines, as they were called, were also able to block only some of the actions of histamine. These discrepancies in the spectrum of activity of the antihistamine and antiadrenaline compounds led to the development, in the last twenty years, of a further series of antagonists (see later) so that now all the actions of adrenaline and histamine can be annulled if necessary.

Finally, Dale found a new substance, which he identified as acetylcholine, in one of his ergot extracts. Again, he dis-

[4] Anaphylactic shock can result from non-protein drugs which have combined with a protein in the body to form an antigen; penicillin does this and kills about twenty people a year in the UK as a result.

covered some fascinating differences: he found that acetylcholine had two distinct types of action. One type could be paralysed by atropine and the other type by nicotine. As with ergometrine, many years had to elapse before acetylcholine was also shown to occur in mammalian tissues and his demonstration of the selective blocking actions of atropine and nicotine played a major part in understanding the physiological function of acetylcholine.

Indeed, Dale had a central role in establishing what we now refer to as the Chemical Theory of Nervous Transmission. When impulses travel along the nerve fibres which pass between brain and muscles, they release, at the end of the nerve, the contents of millions of tiny vesicles, each of them having contained a few thousand molecules of acetylcholine. These molecules of acetylcholine convey the 'information' from nerve ending to muscle fibre and initiate its contraction. Drugs having actions like nicotine, including the arrow poison curare, can annul this action of acetylcholine and produce muscular paralysis. However, when acetylcholine is released at nerve endings in certain organs such as the heart and blood vessels, atropine but not curare is able to block this action.

How does it come about that drugs can pick and choose in this way? How is it that foreign substances can produce such selective actions? Can we learn the rules so that we could produce new selective actions at will? To see the outline of an answer to these questions, we must look at the inner workings of ourselves and related mammals more closely, and this involves considering technicalities of molecules, enzymes and receptors.

Living things are chemical machines which get their energy by burning up (metabolizing) sugars. Sugars are difficult to store in tissues and they are converted into fats which constitute the main fuel store. However, very large molecules (proteins) are used in the structure of tissues from cell walls to skin and bone, the contraction of muscles and the secretions of glands, the transport of oxygen and vitamins in blood, the protection by antibodies, the manufacture (synthesis) of every piece and component of cells and the controlled release of energy from sugars and fats. Proteins are made by joining a large number of small molecules, amino acids, into long chains called polypeptides and there are usually several polypeptide sub-units in each protein. Although there are only 20 primary amino acids, they are arranged in a precise order in each particular protein (determined by other proteins, of course, the genes). The fixed order of the sequence of amino acids in proteins allows these few amino acids to be the basis of everything from viruses to man. A little mental arithmetic informs us that 20 amino acids can be arranged in 2,400,000,000,000,000 different ways and, when we know that each protein may contain several thousand amino acids we can begin, just begin, to appreciate the complex beauty of living things. However, the real beauty of the proteins lies not so much in their strict sequence of amino acids as in their predetermined three-dimensional structure, that is the way the chain of amino acids arranges itself in space like a skein of wool and the way the polypeptide sub-units dovetail into each other. The arrangement is precise but flexible for the sub-units can adjust their position in a limited way, backwards and forwards.

The three-dimensional arrangement and the relative movement of sub-units provide the basis of the catalytic function of proteins. Protein catalysts are called enzymes and catalysis is the facilitation of chemical reactions; but an essential feature of a catalyst is that it is not itself structurally altered when it facilitates the marriage of two other molecules; like the priest catalyst after completing one marriage ceremony, he is free to do it again and again indefinitely! Imagine two species of molecules mixed in a solution which, though they are capable of joining together to form a new third species of molecules, are disinclined to do so. Like all molecules they are dashing about at high speed in a totally random way. When they bump into each other the energy of motion making them tend to spin away again, like colliding billiard balls, is greater than the energy needed to join them together so that not many new molecules are formed. Now add some enzyme which is suitably adapted to catalyse this reaction, i.e. on the surface of the enzyme there is a region, usually a narrow cleft, called the active site, which is adapted in a reciprocal or inverse way to the two 'unwilling' molecules. If one of the molecules gets into the cleft the fit is so precise and snug that it is 'disinclined' to leave. If the other molecule also gets into its (adjacent) site then for a brief moment their vigorous motion is stilled and chemical union can occur. If, now, a third molecule is added to the mixture which also has affinity for the active site, that is it can fit into one of the sites, but which is incapable of forming a chemical union with the other molecule, then the catalytic function of the enzyme will be blocked. This third molecule is a competitive inhibitor (antagonist) of the enzyme.

Many useful drugs act as enzyme inhibitors. Gout is due to excessive formation of uric acid in the body so that solid crystals of sodium urate form in the tissues, particularly in the joints, causing extremely severe pain. Uric acid is formed from the precursor substances hypoxanthine and xanthine at the final stages of purine metabolism. The combination of both these bases with oxygen (oxidation) to form uric acid is catalysed by the enzyme xanthine oxidase. Inhibition of this enzyme will thus slow down the synthesis of uric acid. Allopurinol (Zyloric) is chemically almost identical to hypoxanthine; a carbon and a nitrogen atom are simply transposed in one of the structural rings. But that is enough. Allopurinol has affinity for the active site of xanthine oxidase but since the enzyme fails to combine it with oxygen (oxidation) the enzyme becomes and stays blocked and is prevented from making uric acid. Allopurinol thus successfully prevents attacks of gout. However, the unoxidized precursors xanthine and hypoxanthine now accumulate in the tissues and blood. Fortunately in this case the accumulation of precursors doesn't matter because they are readily eliminated by the kidneys into the urine. Occasionally these substances are present in such large amounts that they crystallize out to form a urinary stone, but drinking extra water and making the urine alkaline with sodium bicarbonate is usually sufficient to keep them soluble and easily eliminated.

As well as causing molecules to marry, enzymes can also cause them to break apart or divorce. Acetylcholine is an ester which can be rapidly broken down to acetic acid and choline by the catalytic enzyme cholinesterase. As described above the acetylcholine is released at the junction between nerve terminals and muscle fibres. As soon as the acetylcholine has stimulated the muscle, the cholinesterase, located on the outside of the muscle fibre, rapidly destroys the transmitter. If the enzyme is inhibited, the effects of nerve impulses become greatly exaggerated and the muscles are thrown into irregular twitching and spasm; if the enzyme is completely inhibited, the muscles become effectively paralysed by the build-up of acetylcholine. The so-called nerve gases (war gases) are capable of forming irreversible chemical bonds with this enzyme and other cholinesterase inhibtors, e.g. malathion, are used as insect poisons. However there are also reversible inhibitors of the enzyme, such as neostigmine, which are valuable for treating myasthenia gravis. In this disease the patient suffers from muscle weakness which is often severe. The muscles behave as though there was not enough acetylcholine being produced. When the cholinesterase is inhibited muscle power returns dramatically because the acetylcholine now stays around longer and gives prolonged stimulation to the muscles. The introduction of treatment by cholinesterase inhibition is described in Chapter 2.

Occasionally, drugs can be used to play tricks on enzymes. The enzyme is offered a drug which closely resembles the molecules which it normally unites or divides (substrates), but which, unlike the unalterable competitive antagonists, is still capable of being handled by the enzyme. The enzyme can be persuaded to make counterfeit molecules! For example the transmitter at sympathetic nerve endings, that is the visceral (involuntary) nerves which adjust our systems for fight, fright or flight, is not adrenaline as Dale thought at the time but an immediate precursor called noradrenaline (norepinephrine). The enzymes which synthesize noradrenaline from DOPA, an earlier amino acid precursor, can also act on administered methylDOPA to produce methylnoradrenaline which has been described as a 'false transmitter' because it is less effective than the normal transmitter. Methyldopa (Aldomet) is used successfully to lower high blood pressure and this effect may be due to the reduction in the effectiveness of the sympathetic nerves which normally constrict blood vessels or to a similar action in the brain.

Most enzymes are not found free in cell fluid but are firmly fixed to cell membranes. There may be several ranks of enzymes so arranged that the products of one reaction immediately become the substrate for the next. Cell membranes are highly specialized structures, made of a mosaic of proteins and fats (lipoproteins), and the movement of molecules and ions across the membrane is strictly regulated. Impedance to the flow of ions gives cell membranes a static charge like an electrified perimeter fence which can be switched on and off as pores in the membrane are opened or closed. This is the mechanism by which cells are sensitive to changes in their environment, the basis of their excitability. Each beat of heart muscle is preceded by a regulated switching off of the cell membrane voltages and the synchronized voltage changes can be detected on the surface of the body with an electrocardiograph. Some drugs used to treat irregular heart beat, the antidysrrhythmics, act on the cell membranes, particularly of the heart, to alter the flux of ionic currents across cell membranes. Lignocaine (Xylocaine) alters the pores through which the sodium ions flow into the heart cells just before each contraction and so can control the speed with which the wave of excitability passes across the heart; it is effective in controlling some disordered rhythms of the heart.

All membranes restrict the movement of other molecules into and out of cells and there are special arrangements to restrict the penetration of substances between other places such as from the blood into the brain and across the placenta into the fetus. To compensate for this, cell membranes are supplied with special chemical pumps, or transport processes, to move particularly valuable substances either way across the membranes. Regulated penetration is particularly important in the kidneys. In the kidneys, blood plasma, that is the fluid non-cellular part of the blood, is first filtered indiscriminately, like filter coffee, into long tubes. The cells lining these tubes have highly-developed systems of transport processes located on their membranes and they actively pick out and return to the blood the molecules they 'want' such as glucose and amino acids and leave behind the 'useless' end-products of protein metabolism such as urea and uric acid. The tubular cells also actively secrete substances, particularly organic acids, including some drugs such as penicillin, directly into the tubular fluid from the blood. Here, where there are specialized chemical processes at work, is another site of drug action.

Penicillin is an organic acid and is eliminated at high speed mainly because it is secreted out of the body by the tubular cells of the kidney. In the early days of penicillin development, when it was extremely expensive to make, this represented a waste of valuable drug. Even today when penicillin is quite cheap to make, rapid elimination by the kidneys can make it difficult to keep the blood levels high enough to treat serious diseases such as bacterial infection of the heart or gonorrhoea when the need is to make a simple massive dose of drug last as long as possible. The answer was found in drugs such as probenecid (Benemid). Probenecid is also an organic acid and competes for the same secretory process as used by penicillin so that the elimination of penicillin is impeded by competition and usefully higher blood levels of drug are attained.

The cell membrane is also the point at which one cell receives chemical messages from other cells. We have already seen how noradrenaline and acetylcholine act as neurotransmitters – released from nerve ends and causing the responding cells, e.g. muscles, to contract. Histamine has been seen to link invading foreign proteins with blood vessels and other tissues. However we now know that there are many, probably thousands, of chemical regulators in the body. The chemical structure of some of these is known and where they are distributed to all cells in the body by the blood rather than released strictly localized to the site of action, they are classed as hormones. The sex hormones, oestradiol and androsterone, are examples, so is triiodothyronine, the thyroid hormone, and insulin which comes from the pancreas. Others are less clearly established, but the existence of numerous chemical regulators to orchestrate the activities of the millions of cells in our bodies is no longer doubted. How does any one cell know what is going on if it is being bombarded by large numbers of different regulators?

Receptors provide the answer. Each chemical regulator has built into its conformation and chemical properties some specific piece of biological information. For that information to be received by a cell the information has to be decoded in the same kind of way that a radio receiver decodes radio waves that it is tuned to receive and no others. A receptor has some similarity to the active site on an enzyme, that is a macromolecular site which shows chemical complementarity in its spatial arrangement and distribution of electronic charges, to the corresponding hormone. However, whereas at an enzyme the substrate is chemically altered and the enzyme remains unchanged, at a receptor the hormone is not altered but the interaction changes the receptor. Changes in the conformation and charge distribution at a receptor then trigger off some predetermined change in cellular activity.

Receptors, like enzymes, are also common sites for drugs to act. After all, both of these sites are designed to be the basis for selective chemical effects in physiology and, if drugs happen to contain enough of the recognizable chemical information, they will be able to deceive the body's own selective machinery. Just as enzyme inhibitors (allopurinol for example) are often closely related chemically to the normal substrate, so receptor antagonists are often closely related chemically to the natural hormone. Knowledge about the physiological function of a specified hormone/receptor system can be used to guess what the properties of a new interfering substance (antagonist) might be. There are many examples of this kind of speculation but here is an example which led to the development of propranolol (Inderal) which is valuable in heart disease and high blood pressure.

Man can live for a few months without food and for a few days without water but even a few minutes without air and oxygen destroys him. Survival depends on how much food, water and oxygen is stored in the body and not much oxygen can be held in blood, the main oxygen store. To hoard a day's supply of oxygen, about 3,000 pints (1,710 litres) of blood or more than 20 times the body weight would be needed; the normal blood volume is about 10 pints (5.5 litres).

When the oxygen supply fails, the heart is an early casualty. Oxygen is supplied to the heart muscle, by arteries through which blood flows mainly during the brief pause between beats, and this delivery is so vital that the heart has its own special blood supply, the coronary arteries. Without oxygen the heart muscle first fails to beat, then dies; the coronary arteries are the heart's own life line.

The heart responds to an increase in bodily activity, be it during exercise or excitement, by beating faster and by pumping more powerfully. The increased force and rate of beating is due to noradrenaline being released at special (sympathetic) nerve endings in the heart fibres. To do this extra work the heart must have more oxygen, and so the coronary arteries must respond by delivering blood faster. Healthy arteries do this, like water taps, by widening the bore. However, diseased arteries have swellings in their inner linings which narrow the bore and so the blood flow cannot increase to meet the demand; if the pipe is furred up, opening the tap wider no longer increases flow. The first sign of trouble that the patient experiences is when the coronary arteries fail to deliver enough blood and oxygen to match the needs of the heart when it is working harder, as during exercise. At the critical point in oxygen delivery, when demand exceeds supply, there is pain, which may be severe – angina pectoris. The muscle may recover when the exercise is stopped by the pain so the heart work is reduced to a level which the coronary arteries can sustain, but the patient's activity is now limited. However, part of the muscle may become damaged beyond repair. This is a myocardial infarct and the cause of 'heart attacks'. After a substantial infarct adequate pumping can still be maintained by the undamaged areas of the muscle provided that enough noradrenaline is secreted at the nerve endings in the heart. The irony of a heart infarct is that the level of stimulation by noradrenaline which is needed to maintain adequate pumping also increases the likelihood that abnormal stimulation of the heart occurs at the boundary between normal and damaged muscle. This abnormal stimulation can wreck coordinated beating of the heart – the wall of the heart becomes a twitching mass of unsynchronized contractions and it suddenly ceases to be an effective pump. This is called fibrillation and usually means sudden death, though prompt application of an electric shock from a 'defibrillator' machine may restore normal rhythm.

Traditionally, angina pectoris has been treated with nitrates and infarction with rest and analgesics. A patient taking nitrates felt warm and flushed in the face and everyone assumed that a similar dilatation of blood vessels occurred in the heart so that more blood could be delivered. A big search went on for drugs which would be better dilators of coronary blood vessels, more selective and longer-lasting, and the search was fairly successful. The newer drugs increased coronary blood flow all right but they often failed to prevent or relieve angina pectoris! Probably there was nothing mysterious about this: diseased arteries cannot dilate as well as healthy ones and the drug actions on blood vessels which tend to increase oxygen supply to the heart also, by inducing nervous reflex changes, act indirectly on heart muscle to increase oxygen demand. If we cannot effectively increase oxygen supply by drugs, why not try to reduce the heart's demand for oxygen? This is what happens anyway when a man with angina pectoris stops for a rest or the patient with an infarct is immobilized in bed. The trouble is that stimulation of the heart by noradrenaline, which mainly determines the heart's demand for oxygen, is only partly controlled by physical exercise – excitement, fear, pain and even lack of physical fitness also promote stimulation of the heart. Physical rest is not enough. Hence the suggestion; why not look for drugs which would prevent noradrenaline acting on the heart as a way of controlling the heart's demand for oxygen?

The noradrenaline receptors are the special chemical sites on heart muscle cells which first recognize and combine with noradrenaline and then trigger the changes in cellular enzymes which make the heart beat faster and more strongly. Propranolol has been found to be a drug which is recognized and bound by the heart's noradrenaline receptors but which not only fails itself to trigger the usual changes in enzyme activity but also, by occupying the receptor, prevents noradrenaline from doing so. This property of propranolol might have been enough to make it useful but it was found to have an additional property which was crucial. The noradrenaline receptors in blood vessels appear to be different from those in the heart. Those in the blood vessels are now classified as mostly alpha-adrenoceptors and propranolol appears to be a selective antagonist of the beta-adrenoceptors found in heart muscle. This means the propranolol interferes with the changes in the heart which occur during exercise or emotion without significantly interfering with the nervous control of the blood vessels. During exercise, the noradrenaline-secreting nerves which supply blood vessels shunt the blood away from skin and abdominal organs and increase the supply to the muscles; this action is not altered by propranolol because beta-adrenoceptors are not involved.

When patients with coronary artery disease are treated with propranolol they are able to do more work without pain and they get short-term relief. However, there is also evidence that long-term blockade of beta-adrenoceptors increases life-expectancy. An unexpected bonus has been the clinical finding that propranolol is an effective treatment for high blood pressure. If this action, as seems likely, is also due to propranolol's capacity to moderate heart work and output during exercise, new light may be thrown on the origin of this widespread disease.

Here is a drug, then, which not only brings relief to sick people but also is valuable in helping us to understand the function of noradrenaline and related hormones in health and disease. This is one of the most important points about drugs today. They do more than bring relief; they are now also important tools in medical research, helping us to understand the nature of disease.

Histamine gives another example of this double use of new drugs. The beta-blockers were discovered after it was found that the early antagonists, the alpha-blockers, were unable to prevent the heart responding to adrenaline. New histamine blockers were discovered after it was found that the old antihistamines were unable to prevent the glands in the stomach, the gastric glands, responding to histamine. Gastric glands secrete hydrochloric acid which contrary to popular belief, is probably less concerned with digestion than with protecting us by sterilizing the upper gut; the incidence of tuberculosis, for example, is higher in people who are unable to secrete acid. Every time we eat, this acid secretion in the stomach is switched on. Some people secrete too much acid either because the stimulus is too strong or perhaps because there is a fault in the mechanism which switches the secretion off once digestion is complete. Either way, excess secretion of acid is associated with ulceration in the stomach and/or duodenum, the adjacent piece of the gut. These ulcers (peptic ulcers) can either make life miserable through pain and indigestion or they may lead to the serious, even lethal, complications of severe bleeding or perforation when the stomach contents leak into the peritoneal space and produce peritonitis. Surgery can excise the glands, removing the ability to secrete acid, or cut the nerves, removing the stimulus to secrete. But these are major operations and more than one in two hundred patients dies as a result.

The nerves which the surgeon cuts secrete acetylcholine at their terminals so that atropine, which is a competitive antagonist to acetylcholine, should be able to achieve the same effect as surgery. Atropine and related drugs have been used to treat peptic ulcers for many years but the results have been disappointing to patient and doctor alike. Doses of atropine which would be needed to reduce acid secretion cause blurred vision, a distressingly dry mouth and trouble in emptying the bladder. Atropine also blocks the nerves going to the muscle in the wall of the stomach so that the emptying of the stomach contents is delayed and prolonged and this might do as much harm as the reduced acid would do good. Atropine just isn't selective enough, not nearly as selective as surgery.

Besides acetylcholine two other substances are found in the stomach which are powerful stimulants of gastric secretion – histamine and gastrin. Gastrin, a polypeptide, released by food from another part of the gut, is the main gastric hormone for controlling gastric secretion. Gastrin reaches its receptors on cells in the gastric mucosa indirectly via the blood. Gastrin stimulates the secretion of digestive enzymes as well as acid. Histamine is made from a single amino acid (histidine) and is concentrated in the region of the acid-secreting cells. Histamine only stimulates acid secretion. Some investigators believe that gastrin stimulates acid secretion indirectly by releasing histamine locally from its storage sites.

Just as noradrenaline acts on two different kinds of receptors so too does histamine. The histamine receptors are identified as H_1- and H_2-types. The antihistamines which we take for hay fever block the H_1-receptors. A few years ago new antagonists were found which could block the H_2-receptors. One of these H_2-receptor antagonists, called cimetidine (Tagamet), is now being used clinically. Although cimetidine is a competitive antagonist of histamine, the effects of gastrin are also suppressed. This could be good news for people with peptic ulcers because gastric acid secretion can now be reduced in a very selective way. More patients can now get the benefit of rapid healing of their ulcers than they could with the previous treatment with drugs which blocked the effects of acetylcholine. They also have the chance of avoiding the serious implications of abdominal surgery. But we do not yet know whether cimetidine has any serious unpredicted unpleasant effects.

Medical scientists have also got a new tool for probing

into the function of histamine. It is possible to think of histamine having a protective function in inflammation and tissue repair, even acid secretion can be seen as part of a protective system. But the puzzling area is the presence of histamine in the brain. Histamine is manufactured in the brain and its function is quite unknown. However, now that we can classify histamine receptors by using drugs like cimetidine some progress is likely and maybe this work will lead to new types of drugs for treating mental disorder.

More and more, we are understanding how drugs make use of the body's own control machinery – receptors, hormones, transport processes, binding sites and so on – to produce selective actions. This understanding gives us a good chance, in the future, of producing many more entirely new drugs which will increase the number of people who can benefit from modern medicine.

However, no matter how skilled we become at making more selective and effective drugs, we will never escape from the problem of drug toxicity. This is an axiom, not an argument. Interaction between a drug and its elective site of action is determined by its goodness-of-fit for the active site plus the likelihood that random molecular motion will bring a molecule into contact with that site. The likelihood of such a molecular encounter is mainly determined by the concentration of molecules. Where a molecular species has high affinity for a site, a low concentration of molecules will achieve effective interaction. But as the concentration is increased, effective interaction may begin to take place at lower affinity sites and new actions, perhaps unwanted and even damaging ones, can then occur. This will be true whether the molecule is natural (hormone) or foreign (drug). A polypeptide hormone secreted by the pituitary gland regulates the water content of the body by controlling its reabsorption in the kidney; if, however large unphysiological doses are given into a vein, a new action, constriction of the blood vessels, appears; even the blood vessels to the heart, the coronary arteries, constrict and a large enough dose can kill an animal by stopping the heart. The latter action was discovered first and the hormone was called vasopressin; the former action was discovered later and so it is now called the antidiuretic hormone. All kinds of hormones and chemical regulators in the human body, such as insulin, histamine, vitamin D, can be lethal when used as a drug and given in overdose.

Except for suicides, the answer to overdose toxicity lies in careful prescribing; the prescriber should give as little of a drug as is necessary to produce the desired effect and carefully monitor his patients.

5. Discovery of new drugs

There are innumerable complex and potentially useful substances found in nature, made by animals, plants, bacteria and fungi. Some are themselves useful medicines, others can be used as a starting point by the modern synthetic chemist who also makes completely new substances that have never hitherto existed.

Until the end of the nineteenth century the discovery of drugs was a matter of chance and serendipity. It can be illustrated by *the history of chemotherapy*, i.e. the treatment of parasitic infections in which the parasites (e.g. bacteria, protozoa, fungi, worms) are destroyed or removed without injuring the host.

Chemotherapy has been practised empirically since ancient times. The Ancient Greeks used male fern (Filix mas) and the Aztecs chenopodium (oil of American wormseed) to eliminate intestinal worms. The Ancient Hindus treated leprosy with chaulmoogra oil (from seeds of Hydnocarpus); there are numerous other examples. For hundreds of years moulds (e.g. penicilliums) have been applied to wounds, but, despite the introduction of mercury as a treatment for syphilis (sixteenth century), and the use of cinchona bark against malaria (seventeenth century), the history of modern rational chemotherapy does not begin until the late nineteenth century.

With the knowledge of bacterial and protozoal causation of diseases and the development of techniques for infecting laboratory animals, scientific therapeutic experiments could be performed. These animal experiments were not subject to the restrictions of clinical therapeutics, toxicity could be risked, and large numbers of infections treated under controlled conditions. In addition, acceptance of archaic authority and belief in magic were on the wane and a scientific approach to medical problems was becoming less rare.

It is not surprising that the differential staining of tissues and bacteria by dyes used for microscopical techniques should have been the basis of early chemotherapeutic research, for it was an obvious instance of chemicals affecting parasite and host differently and gave hope of usefully selective toxicity, which is the objective of drug therapy. Aniline dyes were used for staining and, when it was shown that these dyes could also kill bacteria, Ehrlich,[1] already interested in the differential staining of leucocytes, tried the effect of dyes on infected experimental animals. In 1891 he cured experimental malaria in guinea pigs with methylene blue, but it was less effective than quinine. In 1904 he controlled trypanosome (African sleeping sickness) infections in mice with another dye, trypan red, but it was ineffective in other species.

Ehrlich thus developed the idea of 'chemotherapy' and he invented the word. In 1906 he wrote:

'In order to use chemotherapy successfully we must search for substances which have an affinity for the cells of the parasites and a power of killing them greater than the damage such substances cause to the organism itself, so that the destruction of the parasite will be possible without seriously hurting the organism. This means we must strike the parasites and the parasites only, if possible, and to do this we must learn to aim, learn to aim with chemical substances!'[2]

Or, as a modern microbiologist has put it in reverse, formaldehyde 'admittedly will fix the patient's bacteria, but will also fix the patient'.[3]

Knowledge of the relationship between chemical structure and pharmacological action (i.e. learning to aim with chemicals) has steadily increased until at last it is being effectively applied to the development of new drugs.

By 1906 it was clear that chemotherapy was a practical proposition and not the fantasy that eminent contemporaries declared it. Inorganic arsenic had been shown to clear trypanosomes from the blood of infected horses and an organic

[1] Paul Ehrlich (1854-1915), one of the most important medical scientists ever: a variety of other important contributions: Frankfurt, Germany.

[2] Marquardt, M. (1949), *Paul Ehrlich*, Heinemann.

[3] Jawetz, E. (1963), *British Medical Journal*, 2, 951.

arsenical had been used successfully on man. This inspired Ehrlich to make and test further compounds. His efforts resulted in the introduction of arsphenamine (Salvarsan) for the treatment of syphilis and it was soon followed by neo-arsphenamine (Neosalvarsan) which was widely used until 1945 when it was superseded by pencillin.

After neoarsphenamine there was a lull. Then the anti-malarials pamaquin and mepacrine were developed from dyes and in 1935 the first sulphonamide linked with a dye (Prontosil), was introduced as a result of empirical experiments by Domagk.[4]

The results obtained with sulphonamides in puerperal sepsis (infection of the genital tract after childbirth), pneumonia and meningitis were dramatic and caused a reorientation of medical thought. Until then chemotherapy had been virtually confined to protozoa and worms, spirochaetes (syphilis) being considered as a special case. To kill 'ordinary' pyogenic bacteria (streptococci, staphylococci, etc.) in the body had seemed impossible.

In 1928, seven years before the discovery of the sulphonamides, Fleming[5] whilst studying staphylococcal variants found one of his culture plates contaminated with a fungus which destroyed surrounding bacterial colonies. This accidental rediscovery of the long-known ability of penicillin fungi to suppress the growth of *in vitro* bacterial cultures was now followed up. Fleming investigated the properties of 'mould broth filtrates' which, for brevity, he named 'penicillin'. He described penicillin as an antiseptic more powerful than phenol (carbolic acid) which yet could safely be applied to the tissues. The name 'penicillin' has since applied to the pure antibiotic substance (an antibiotic is a substance produced by living organisms that also at high dilution kills organisms).

Attempts to isolate penicillin from the crude preparations were made, but lack of appreciation of its potentialities as well as the difficulty of preparing enough for experiments caused it to be put aside as a curiosity, although Fleming used it in his laboratory as a method of differentiating

[4] Gerhard Domagk (1895-   ), biochemist, Germany.
[5] Alexander Fleming (1881-1955), microbiologist, London, discoverer of penicillin.

bacterial cultures throughout the 1930s.

In 1939, principally as an academic exercise, Chain[6] and Florey[7] in Oxford undertook a new investigation of anti-biotics. They prepared penicillin, discovered that it was effective if introduced into the blood so that it was carried throughout the body, as well as when applied to local surface infections, in mice, and confirmed its remarkable lack of toxicity.

The importance of this discovery for a nation at war was obvious to these workers but the time, July 1940, was un-propitious, for Britain was being bombarded from the sky with increasing vigour. It was necessary to manufacture penicillin in the Oxford University Pathology Laboratory where enough was made to start a small clinical trial in 1941. The results appeared good and it was clear that penicillin might have military importance, but because of the war large-scale production in Britain was not possible. The USA was still at peace, so arrangements were made for the pro-duction of penicillin there. Ample supplies were available to treat casualties in the latter part of the war.

Since 1939 large programmes of screening fungi and bacteria for antibiotic production have been conducted. The first success was the isolation of streptomycin from a soil organism (streptomyces) and this was followed by the tetra-cyclines, erythromycin and others. Simultaneously there have been developments in synthetic agents, especially against tuberculosis and tropical diseases, including malaria, leprosy and amoebic dysentery. That nothing is beneath the notice of some investigators is illustrated by the discovery of anti-bacterial substances in the anal gland secretion of the Argentine ant and in the faeces of blow-fly larvae.

Most important infective diseases are now, to some extent at least, treatable. Prominent exceptions include small viruses and South American trypanosomiasis. The small viruses pre-sent a special problem in that they enter host cells and use host mechanisms to multiply there, so that selective chemical attack is specially difficult, though progress is being made. In any case the peak of virus multiplication precedes symp-toms, i.e. by the time you know you have got influenza

[6] E. B. Chain (1906-   ), biochemist, Oxford, Rome, London.
[7] H. W. Florey (1898-1968), pathologist, Oxford.

most of the damage has been done already, so cure presents great problems. However substances capable of preventing the virus entering the host cells also exist and these offer prospects of effective prevention.

DRUG RESEARCH

Most new drugs are developed in industrial rather than in academic laboratories. These two kinds of laboratory are complementary, having important, though different, approaches, the 'organized opportunism' of the industrial and the 'knowledge for its own sake' of the academic laboratory. The academic workers are often fired with interest to use the largely empirical discoveries of the industrialists as tools to explore fundamental mechanisms. The rational development of new drugs by industry is easier where the fundamental biochemical nature of normal and diseased processes, more widely, though not exclusively, studied in academic laboratories is understood; for example the development of antihistamines depended on knowledge that histamine was released in the body and was a causative factor in urticaria and hay fever; the efficacy of allopurinol in gout could be predicted from knowledge of the path of synthesis of uric acid in the body. A cure for human cancer is more likely to be found if details of the biochemistry of malignant and normal cells are known, than it is by empirically testing tens of thousands of chemicals selected at random or because they are related to existing relatively unselective and inefficient drugs. Drugs are tested in animals in which cancer has been artificially induced or which have been bred to have a high incidence of the disease, as well as in tissue culture.

'The most frequent purpose of research in the drug industry can be stated simply; it is to discover profitable drugs. For a drug to be profitable it should be both useful and safe, properties that are determined eventually by the clinician. The task of the pharmacologist is to predict these properties from animal experiments, within the limitations imposed by availability of facilities and staff. This must be done in such a way that the possibility of missing a useful drug is minimized; in other words, the "screening" programme must be efficient.'[8]

The greatest difficulties for the laboratory pharmacologist lie in designing his animal experiments to yield the maximum information from a relatively few animals and to be relevant to human physiology and disease. It is, for example, particularly difficult to design animal experiments to test drugs for their possible efficacy in human mental disorders, but relatively easy to test them for anticoagulant effects because animal and human blood clots by similar mechanisms and because measurement of clotting is easy.

New drugs may be sought in a number of ways: most new drugs are developed from old drugs. The old drug is used as a standard of comparison in an animal test and it is also used as the starting point for the medicinal chemist. Imagine there is a drug which is known to be valuable in the treatment of mental depression – an antidepressant. There is no way of producing psychological depression in animals. However, academic pharmacologists find that the antidepressant will reverse the actions of reserpine in experimental animals – a drug known to produce severe mental depression and even suicide in man. Reserpine produces physical depression, and immobility, in animals and so reserpine-reversal in mice is used as a screening test, in the hope that this action in mice will correlate with the desired therapeutic action which the parent antidepressant compound has in man. A cycle of chemical modification, screening test, evaluation and then a new chemical modification will usually lead to new drugs which are more active, less toxic or easier to use than the original one.

This is an empirical method but it is sound and effective even if there is no great novelty at the end. The 'molecular roulette' pejorative does not apply to this procedure. A great deal of imaginative skill and experience is used by the medicinal chemist when he moves systematically from parent-compound to new drug. Any pressure to reduce this kind of industrial research because of notions of repetition and 'me-tooism' would, we believe, be foolish and rob us

⁸ Vane, J. R. (1964), in *Evaluation of Drug Activities,* eds. Laurence, D. R., Bacharach, A. L., Academic Press.

of some of our best chances to get maximally effective medication. Of course, commercial marketing practices can sometimes obscure the best features of this work by promoting, often with official acquiescence, meretricious developments which only confuse and complicate therapeutics.

The above approach starts from a known compound and has a clear therapeutic objective. However there is a closely-related approach to finding new drugs which has got neither of these merits. Often called 'random-screening', this approach uses a whole battery of different animal tests. These often begin with a simple 'observational' test of animal behaviour. In this several doses of the compound are given to groups of mice, and their behaviour is monitored by trained observers or automatic apparatus, activity, temperature, heart and respiratory rates, etc., are recorded and compared with undosed control groups. All changes or lack of changes are registered on special forms or fed into a computer which provides a 'profile' of activity.

This profile is examined and is compared with the profiles of standard drugs which, with inert control injections, are also put through the test system from time to time to check it for reliability and sensitivity. Of course, observers must always be kept ignorant of what the animals have received, for they (the observers) are subject to natural human bias from their expectations, mood, alertness, etc.

It is claimed that this kind of test, which is now highly refined, can detect the following types of drugs: sedative, hypnotic, tranquillizer, psychic stimulant, muscle relaxant, analgesic, convulsant, neuromuscular-blocking, atropine-like, ganglion-blocking, sympathomimetic, antipyretic, vasodilator, acetylcholine-like.

Any such screening test is a compromise based on the imagined risk of missing useful drugs and the need for simplicity and speed. No one knows whether more valuable drugs have been missed than have been found.

Any compound thought to be of interest in this 'primary screen' is then subjected to more detailed pharmacological and sometimes biochemical study devised in the light of the initial results. This investigation may be done on whole animals with recording of various physiological functions and on isolated tissues *in vitro*. Several species of animal will be used, generally chosen from mice, rats, cats and dogs, and sometimes guinea pigs and rabbits.

Although there is a certain amount of wishful thinking in random screening, this faculty is most obvious when experimental diseases are used for screening. The experimental diseases may be high blood pressure, stomach ulcers, arthritis or convulsions: all these animal tests have in common a superficial resemblance to certain human diseases but differ from them in that, unlike the actual disease, the 'cause' of them in the experimental animals is known. These disease models give the medicinal chemist no guidance for his starting point so that finding an entirely novel drug by this approach is exceedingly difficult.

Finally, there is a style of new drug research which starts with physiological control processes and sets out to find substances which can annul or mimic them. The medicinal chemist starts with a known hormone or substance and the pharmacologist can evaluate any new compounds on a precisely defined biological test. Chemicals are made in the light of detailed knowledge of the biological process with which it is wished to interfere, whether this be bacterial or cancer growth or brain metabolism. Research commonly takes the form of making slight chemical variants of natural metabolites and presenting these to the cell it is wished to affect 'in the hope that the forgeries will upset its utilization of the true metabolite'.[9] This way is more likely than the others to introduce real novelty into therapeutics but there are no *a priori* grounds for being sure that the well-defined tool developed to interfere in physiological processes will also be useful in the treatment of human diseases. The empirical element is transferred from the laboratory to the clinic, i.e. we have a drug looking for a disease. Oddly enough this process has shown some remarkable successes (see Chapter 4).

The above account may suggest that drugs are always discovered by a planned approach, however unimaginative. But an important factor in drug discovery, namely luck, has to be mentioned. Whilst luck cannot, obviously, be a formally planned aspect of drug research, yet the research can be conducted in such a way that the unexpected, unpredicted event will be observed, discussed and followed up. For

[9] Vane, J. R. (1964), op. cit.

example the shrewd observation and exploration of events occurring in the clinic has led to the development of anti-depressants from antituberculosis drugs: of antidiabetics and diuretics from antibacterial sulphonamides: of anti-hypertensive treatment by drugs prescribed for angina pectoris.

As well as testing the effects of graded single doses, chronic pharmacological studies with regular dosage for days or weeks are sometimes needed, for there are drugs that, as well as acutely altering some bodily functions, also change others more slowly (e.g. some tranquillizers and drugs for high blood pressure; oral contraceptives), and many drugs are now given to man for years.

Studies of what happens to the drug in the body (absorption, distribution, elimination) should also be undertaken in animals; and when correlated with preliminary studies in man they can often enhance prediction.

These pharmacological studies are integrated with those of the toxicologist to build up a picture of the unwanted as well as the wanted drug effects. Some information on toxicity will generally have been got during the initial pharmacological testing, and this is extended by the toxicologist's special investigations.

TOXICITY TESTING

All drugs are poisons and the task of the toxicologist is to find out how they act in animals, often using very high doses, and to give an opinion on the significance of his data in relation to risks likely to be run by human beings receiving the drug. This will remain a nearly impossible task until biochemical explanations of all effects can be provided. The toxicologist is in an unenviable position. When a useful drug is safely introduced he is considered to have done no more than his duty. When an accident occurs he is invited to explain how this failure of prediction came about. When he predicts that a chemical is unsafe in a major way for man, his prediction is never tested. *Acute toxicity testing* aims first at establishing what is unsuitably called the therapeutic index or ratio. This concept was devised by Ehrlich as maximum tolerated dose/minimum curative dose to give some indication of the safety of antimicrobial drugs. In clinical practice the index is never calculated, for the data are not available in a suitable form, especially for drugs used over long periods. However, the concept embodies a sensible way of thinking about drugs, i.e. safety in relation to efficacy.

In a drug development laboratory practical use can be made of a modification of this concept provided it is recognized that, as with all animal data, it cannot be arbitrarily transferred to man. The therapeutic index for animals is nowadays calculated as the ratio LD_{50}/ED_{50}, i.e. the dose that is lethal to 50% of animals (LD_{50}) divided by the dose that has the desired effect in 50% of animals (ED_{50}).

But it is more important to discover *how* the compound acts as a poison and this may need microscopical and biochemical studies with repeated, or chronic, administration.

Short-term (subacute) and long-term (chronic) toxicity testing involves giving the compound daily for between one week and the lifetime of the animals, generally rats and dogs. Except for testing for carcinogenesis, little is generally gained by exceeding six months' regular administration at several doses. Duration of the tests and their exact nature will differ widely according to whether a drug may be given once or a few times (e.g. general anaesthetic) or continuously for years (e.g. antiepileptic).

Generally a drug is given daily and the appearance, activity, food intake, growth and reproductive ability in groups of animals on different doses are observed. Biochemical studies (urine, blood, etc.) are commonly done and microscopic examination of most tissues, but especially blood, bone marrow, liver and kidneys, are done in animals that die as well as in sample animals killed at intervals during the test.

Species differences between animals and between animals and man are the source of difficult problems of interpretation. Perhaps the most famous species difference is the lethal bleeding from the intestine of guinea pigs following penicillin administration (due to an effect on the gut bacteria on which vegetarian species rely to break down cellulose) and its negligible toxicity to non-herbivores, including man.

Fortunately such differences of the effect of a drug on the body (pharmacodynamics) are less common than are differences in the effect of the body on a drug (pharmacokinetics). Occasionally gross differences in rate or path of metabolism may make chronic toxicity studies undertaken to predict toxicity to man misleading.

The special problems of testing for adverse effects on the fetus and for causation of cancer or genetic changes have been mentioned in an earlier chapter.

EXPERIMENTS IN ANIMALS

New drugs are investigated in animals both for the desired (therapeutic) effects and for the undesired (toxic) effects. Many tests are done on unconscious anaesthetized animals and many on isolated organs of animals killed 'humanely'. But it is hard to doubt that, especially in toxicity testing, a lot of suffering is caused to conscious animals.

All this would be totally unjustified if results useful to man could not be obtained. In many known respects animals are similar to man, but in some respects they are not.

It would be hypocritical for a society that tolerates first the mutilation (e.g. castration) and later, after short confined lives, the killing of animals for food – let alone chasing them about the fields to their death or driving them towards lines of gunmen for recreation – to shrink from employing them for maintaining health and life in other ways. At present, in order to begin to decide whether a chemical is a medicine or merely a chemical, either animal experiments (involving whole animals or animal tissues) must be done, or substances of almost totally unknown biological effect must be given to man. Failing either of these, drug therapy must cease to advance. We choose the first course.

As knowledge of basic mechanisms advances, *in vitro* biochemical preparations and tissue cultures may one day allow better prediction of what effect a drug will have in man, but whole animals will still be necessary to determine the final outcome on complex inter-related systems.

Animals are also used extensively to test cosmetics, food additives, preservatives which are necessary to allow food to be supplied in big cities, as well as colouring which is unnecessary, chemicals used in industry, etc. Plainly these activities all pose ethical problems.

CONCLUSION

A dominant feature of the problem of finding new drugs to alleviate or cure disease is that of predicting from experiments with chemicals on animals what effect these chemicals will have in man.

As drugs are developed and promoted for long-term use in more and relatively trivial conditions, e.g. minor anxiety or slight high blood pressure, and affluent societies become less and less willing to tolerate small physical or mental discomforts or unhappiness, demanding relief without even minor inconvenience, drug therapy will continue to increase and the problem of demonstrating not only the efficacy, but also the safety of drugs, will grow. Profound knowledge of biochemical mechanisms may some day eliminate risk in the introduction of new drugs, but this is far off. In the meantime failures of prediction will continue to occur. Another disaster as horrible as thalidomide may happen again although, with growth of adequate systems for monitoring possible adverse reactions, it should be on a much smaller scale.

Limited resources of scientific manpower and money will not be used to the best advantage if the public shock over thalidomide is allowed to express itself in governmental regulations requiring a plethora of expensive tests (and toxicity testing is very expensive), of dubious meaning for anything other than the animal concerned, for this would prevent industrial laboratories (whoever controls them) from devoting resources to investigation of fundamental mechanisms of drug action, in the knowledge of which alone lies health with safety.

6. Development of new medicines

When a new chemical considered to be a potentially useful drug has been discovered in tests on animals then the time has come to put it to the test in man.

FIRST CLINICAL TRIAL OF POTENTIAL DRUGS

The clinician has to satisfy himself that the animal laboratory studies are adequate in kind, quality and extent to justify the risk of administering to man a chemical that has hitherto been tried on animals only. He should not allow himself to be convinced too easily. He should only consent to try the chemical on man if there is evidence that existing drugs for the purpose are imperfect, as is, in fact, always the case, so that there is a place for a new one. Ideally he should require some hint that the potential drug has been shown in experimental animals to offer hope of improvement and that the toxicity studies have been meticulous and satisfactory. Failing this, trial on man must be a greater gamble than it ought to be.

However, if these criteria are rigidly insisted on then no doubt useful drugs will be missed. This point has been put cogently:[1] 'It is possible to waste too much time in animal studies before testing a drug in man'; though satisfactory both qualitatively and quantitatively in animals, it may be useless in man solely because its duration of action is too short or too long, so that 'the practice of studying the physiologic disposition of a drug in man only after it is clearly the drug of choice in animals not only may prove short-sighted and time consuming, but also may result in relegating the best drug for man to the shelf for ever more'. Despite

[1] Brodie, B. B. (1962), *Clinical Pharmacology and Therapeutics, 3,* 374.

the undoubted force of this argument, clinical workers may require additional persuasion to try a compound that is not 'the drug of choice in animals'.

The path of the industrial drug developer is a stony, even if sometimes a highly profitable, one. He risks huge sums of money but the clinician, sympathetic though he should be, must ruthlessly resist any trial in man involving any avoidable risks. Whilst the clinician must not demand too much, equally he must not allow commercial pressures to affect his judgement of what is best for the sick.

This account of drug development, largely stressing the difficulties and the imponderables, may be put into perspective by the following figures on the general safety of drugs in relation to accidents and to smoking, in Britain (population 57 million) in one recent year:

> *Deaths due to:*
> therapeutic use of drugs
>
> | | |
> |---|---:|
> | (certified as *prime* cause of death) | 43 |
> | accidents to children | 1,700 |
> | motor vehicle accidents | 7,084 |
> | accidents in the home | 6,000 |
> | lung cancer | |
> | (largely due to smoking) | 28,252 |

Unreliable though these figures may be (doctors understandably avoid certifying their treatment as the principal cause of death if it is at all reasonable to do so), they probably do approximate justice to the relative risks of drug therapy, cars and smoking.

Rational clinical introduction of a potential new drug requires study in four successive stages:
1. The effects of the drug (pharmacodynamics) on healthy volunteers or patients, often in a special clinical laboratory, to determine whether the effects seen in animals occur in man; study of absorption, distribution, metabolism and excretion (pharmacokinetics) proceeds in parallel.
2. Wider use on patients to establish potential therapeutic utility, dosage schedules and some notion of common adverse effects.
3. Formal assessment of its therapeutic merits, compared with those of other remedies, when these exist.

4. Monitoring for adverse reactions as well as therapeutic benefit after general release.

As the number of potential drugs produced increases, the problem of who to test them on grows. Clearly there are three main groups, healthy volunteers, patient volunteers and, rarely, patient non-volunteers. This matter will not be discussed in detail here, but it is relevant to note that some drug actions can be determined on the healthy (anticoagulant, anaesthetic, blood pressure lowering) whereas others cannot (drugs for heart failure or cancer) so that to try the latter on the healthy to obtain data on what happens to the drug in the body (pharmacokinetics) would be to treat man formally as an experimental animal, risking toxicity, however remotely, to obtain information of no benefit to the subject. This is increasingly often done in healthy volunteers and raises the question of what constitutes 'informed' consent, especially if some volunteers are prisoners as is at present the case in at least one country (USA). This procedure may or may not be thought proper.

It is intolerable that a potential new drug should be given to a person who has not been consulted except in the rarest circumstances (advanced mental disease, childhood and in other situations where ability to comprehend is impaired) and here any experiment should have direct therapeutic intent, and not be merely to get information that will advance knowledge and benefit others. If the patient cannot be consulted then his relatives must be.

Considerable problems of ethics arise in testing drugs and it is now usual to require that all such projects be subjected to formal ethical review by an independent committee comprising medical, nursing, legal and lay members. Indeed the Medical Research Council in Britain and equivalent bodies supporting research in the USA require such approval as a condition of making grants for clinical research.

The first two stages of clinical drug development are generally conducted by specialists, but any doctor in hospital or general practice may nowadays find himself concerned with formal clinical evaluation either as a participant or examining reports in order to decide whether to use a drug on his patients.

EXPERIMENTAL THERAPEUTICS

Pickering[2] has written:

'. . . therapeutics is the branch of medicine that, by its very nature, should be experimental. For if we take a patient afflicted with a malady and we alter his conditions of life . . . we are performing an experiment. And if we are scientifically minded we should record the results. Before concluding that the change for better or for worse in the patient is due to the specific treatment employed, we must ascertain . . . whether the result was merely due to the natural history of the disease . . . or whether it was due to some other factor which was necessarily associated with the therapeutic measure in question. And if, as a result of these procedures, we learn that the therapeutic measure employed produces a significant, though not very pronounced improvement, we would experiment with the method, altering dosage or other detail to see if it can be improved. This would seem the procedure to be expected of men with six years of scientific training behind them.

'But it has not been followed. Had it been done we should have gained a fairly precise knowledge of the place of individual methods of therapy in disease, and our efficiency as doctors would have been enormously enhanced.'

There are some who dislike or reject the notion of deliberate experimentation on the sick, feeling that a scientific approach implies an unsympathetic or even a malevolent disposition. They forget that in the past positively harmful treatments have been widely used for many years (e.g. bleeding for pneumonia) though with the the best of motives, because of the lack of recognition of the need, as well as lack of knowledge of the techniques, of scientific evaluation of therapy. It has been pointed out that where the worth of a treatment, new or old, is in doubt, there may be a

[2] Sir George Pickering, FRS (1904–   ), lately Professor of Medicine, St Mary's Hospital, London, Regius Professor of Medicine, Oxford (*Proceedings of the Royal Society of Medicine.* 1949, *42*, 229).

greater obligation to test it critically than to go on prescribing it supported only by habit or wishful thinking.

The choice before the doctor is not whether he should
experiment on his patients, but whether he should do so in
a planned or in a haphazard fashion; whether he should try
to organize his experience so that it is of value to himself
and to others or to follow the notoriously unreliable 'clinical
impression'. To rely on impressions is the less ethical course.

Anyone who thinks he can assess the value of any but the
most dramatically effective treatments by using them on
patients in an uncontrolled fashion has the whole history of
therapeutics against him. It is given to only a few to test a
treatment that radically alters disease and whose efficacy is
obvious with only casual use, and even then details of its
administration will generally need carefully planned studies,
e.g. adrenal steroids in rheumatoid arthritis and asthma,
where benefits can be enormous but where wrong use may
be worse than useless.

Modern scientific techniques uncover the most effective
treatments whilst exposing the smallest numbers to those
that are less effective or even positively harmful; they save
lives, time and money. They are not unethical for they are
only properly used where the relative merits of treatments
are genuinely unknown.

Some patients find it hard to put their confidence in a
doctor who, openly admitting uncertainty, is using two treatments concurrently in order to achieve a true measure of
their relative values. They need the emotional security that
is provided by a doctor who behaves as though he knows,
indeed, who sometimes himself believes he knows, even
though they may rightly suspect that there are others of
equal authority who take an opposite view. The authors of
this book make a point of taking their own illnesses to
colleagues who are prepared to admit ignorance when they,
in fact, don't know.

Though the 'statistical therapeutic comparison' or 'formal
clinical trial', which will be discussed below, is a powerful
tool for advancing therapy, it does not suit every occasion.
Sometimes, as in malaria, there are clinical or laboratory
tests that will rapidly tell whether a treatment is effective,
though they may not provide evidence of a marginal difference between effective drugs, and in tuberculous meningitis

a single recovery was considered adequate evidence of the therapeutic efficacy of streptomycin on a disease with 100% mortality.

NEED FOR STATISTICS

In order to decide whether patients treated in one way are benefited more than those treated in another, there is no possibility of avoiding the use of numbers. The mere statement by a clinician that patients do better with this or that treatment is due to his having formed an opinion that more patients are helped by the treatment he advocates than by other treatments. The opinion is based on numbers, but having omitted to record exactly how many patients have been treated by different methods and having omitted to ensure that the only variable factor affecting the patient was the treatment in question, only a 'clinical impression', instead of facts, can be stated. This is a pity, for progress is delayed when convinced opinions are offered in place of convincing facts. The former, though not necessarily wrong, are unreliable, despite the great assurance with which they are often advanced. This is not to dismiss the anecdotal clinical survey or the case-report, for they tell what can happen, which is useful. Also, formal therapeutic trials are often undertaken because someone has formed an impression which is thought to deserve testing.

A century ago Francis Galton saw this clearly.

'In our general impressions far too great a weight is attached to what is marvellous . . . Experience warns us against it, and the scientific man takes care to base his conclusions upon actual numbers. The human mind is . . . a most imperfect apparatus for the elaboration of general ideas . . . General impressions are never to be trusted. Unfortunately when they are of long standing they become fixed rules of life, and assume a prescriptive right not to be questioned. Consequently, those who are not accustomed to original enquiry entertain a hatred and a horror of statistics. They cannot endure the idea of submitting their sacred impressions to cold-blooded verification. But it is the triumph of scientific men to rise superior to such superstitions, to devise tests by which the value of beliefs may be ascertained, and to feel sufficiently masters of themselves to discard contemptuously whatever may be found untrue . . . the frequent incorrectness of notions derived from general impressions may be assumed . . .'[3]

Statistics tell us of probabilities; reasonable certainty is only obtained when there are several independent studies all reaching similar conclusions; absolute certainty is only attained where there is certain knowledge of mechanisms so that statistics become unnecessary.

THERAPEUTIC TRIAL DESIGN

The aims of a therapeutic trial, not all of which can be attempted on any one occasion, are to decide:
1. whether a treatment is of value,
2. how great its value is (compared with other remedies, if such exist),
3. in what types of patients it is of value,
4. what is the best method of applying the treatment; how often, and in what dosage if it is a drug,
5. what are the disadvantages and dangers of the treatment.

The development of modern techniques of design and analysis of therapeutic trials which allow drugs or other treatments to be evaluated on relatively small numbers of patients is at least as important as the development of many new drugs. This development has occurred largely over the past 30 years though the principles were set down by Claude Bernard[4] in 1864. 'We cannot judge the influence of a remedy on the course and outcome of a disease if we do not previously know the natural course and outcome of the disease . . . To be valid, comparative experiments have therefore to be made at the same time and on as comparable patients as possible. In spite of that, such comparisons still bristle with immense difficulties · which physicians must strive to lessen;

[3] Galton, F. (1879), 'Generic images', *Proceedings of the Royal Institute*: Francis Galton (1822-1911), geneticist, biostatistician.

[4] Claude Bernard (1813-77), French physiologist, one of the greatest medical scientists, author of *Introduction to the Study of Experimental Medicine*.

for comparative experiment is the *sine qua non* of scientific experimental medicine; without it a physician walks at random and becomes the plaything of endless illusions. A physician, who tries a remedy and cures his patients, is inclined to believe that the cure is due to his treatment. Physicians often pride themselves on curing all their patients with a remedy that they use. But the first thing to ask them is whether they have tried doing nothing, i.e. not treating their patients; for how can they otherwise know whether the remedy or nature cured them? . . . We may be subject daily to the greatest illusions about the value of treatment if we do not have recourse to comparative experiment. I shall only recall one recent example concerning the treatment of pneumonia. Comparative experiment showed, in fact, that treatment of pneumonia by bleeding, which was believed most efficacious, is a mere therapeutic illusion.'

Bradford Hill[5] defines the therapeutic trial as

'a carefully, and ethically, designed experiment with the aim of answering some *precisely framed question*. In its most rigorous form it demands *equivalent groups* of patients *concurrently treated* in different ways. These groups are constructed by the *random allocation* of patients to one or other treatment . . . In principle the method is applicable with any disease and any treatment. It may also be applied on any scale; it does not necessarily demand large numbers of patients.'

Of course, now, when there are effective treatments, new treatments are compared against current effective treatments and patients who should be treated are not left untreated, which would be unethical.

EXPERIMENTATION ON MAN

Plainly the development of new treatments involves experimentation on man.

Ethics of human experimentation are of grave concern

⁵ Sir Austin Bradford Hill, FRS (1897-   ), doyen of medical statisticians ('Principles of Medical Statistics', London, *Lancet*, 1977).

to all who use drugs, especially new drugs, and some aspects have already been mentioned.

Human experiments are of two main kinds:

1. *therapeutic:* those that may actually have a beneficial effect or provide information that can be used to help the subject, and

2. *non-therapeutic:* those that provide information that cannot be of direct use to him, though it may advance knowledge in a way useful to other patients present or future.

In practice, experiments often do not fall clearly into one or other group and attempts to lay down codes of behaviour based on the assumption that they do have so far failed to achieve their object of allowing medicine to advance whilst certainly preventing abuse.

Some dislike the word 'experiment' in relation to man, thinking that its mere use implies a degree of impropriety in what is done. It is better, however, that all should recognize the true meaning of the word 'to ascertain or establish by trial',[6] that the benefits of modern medicine derive wholly from experimentation and that some risk, however slight, is inseparable from medical advance. The duty of all doctors lies in ensuring that in their enthusiasm for knowledge, to advance their reputation and career as well as in their desire to help patients in general, they should never allow themselves to put the individual who has sought their aid at any disadvantage, for 'the scientist or physician has no right to choose martyrs for society'.[7] Nowadays it is usual to have formal ethical review of all human experimental programmes by committees that include non-medical representation.

Physicians deal with individuals and have sometimes argued against the statistical therapeutic trial that it does not tell what will happen to any one individual who consults them. This is obviously true, but the knowledge gained from such studies that, with a treatment, $x\%$ recover, $y\%$ improve and $z\%$ are unchanged (and that this result is unlikely to be due to chance), together with details of unwanted effects, provides a better basis for the choice of therapy for individuals than the, often divergent, clinical impressions of doctors.

[6] *Oxford English Dictionary.*

[7] Kety, S., quoted by Beecher, H. K. (1962), *Clinical Pharmacology and Therapeutics, 3,* 141.

It is, of course, only proper to perform a therapeutic trial when the doctor genuinely does not know which treatment is best, and if he is prepared to withdraw individual patients, or to stop the whole trial if at any time he becomes convinced that it is in their interest to do so. A sound guide to ethical conduct is, 'no patient should be worse off as a result of the trial than he might have been otherwise in the hands of a reasonable and competent medical man'.[8]

If it is not known whether one treatment is better than another, then nothing is lost by allotting patients at random to those treatments under test, and it is in everybody's interest that good treatments should be adopted and bad treatments abandoned as soon as possible. It is, of course, more difficult to justify testing a new treatment where existing treatments are fairly good than where they are bad, and this difficulty is likely to grow as medicine advances. With a new drug the situation is generally clear – its efficacy is unknown – but when a drug has been marketed and used for years without proper scientific evaluation so that unsupported claims surround it, then the difficulties of getting true scientific evaluation are multiplied, for 'long years of habitual prescribing based on early and authoritative impressions and optimism confers on a drug qualities of survival which have a high degree of immunity against the disqualifying actions of scientific experiment in man'.[9]

Despite all the technical difficulties and ethical problems we consider that the standard of evaluation of new drugs for efficacy and safety is, at its best, a high one and that accidents and unethical behaviour are very much the exception, though, of course, human nature being what it is, they occur, as do carelessness and incompetence, in this as in any other human activity.

[8] Glaser, E. M. (1964), in *Medical Surveys and Clinical Trials,* ed. Witts, L. J., London, OUP.

[9] Gold, H. (1959), in *Quantitative Methods in Human Pharmacology and Therapeutics,* ed. Laurence, D. R., London, Pergamon.

7. Government control of medicines

Proposals to regulate the availability of medicines are not new. A physician[1] wrote in 1807 that,

'The History of the Materia Medica affords abundant examples of the temporary celebrity, and subsequent neglect, of many of its articles . . . It is greatly to be wished that the eminent bodies appointed to regulate our Pharmacopoeias would deign to take this important subject into their consideration. The really efficacious and useful medicines to be found in the extensive lists that at present form the Materia Medica, might probably be comprised within a comparatively narrow space; and . . . it would in a great degree facilitate the study of this important branch of medicine, were the superabundant articles expunged.'

About 170 years later a Committee on Review of Medicines was set up in the UK to do exactly this.

When the individual consumer cannot judge for himself the quality of a manufactured product and the adequacy of the instructions and information with which the supplier provides him, then it is the job of government to help.

Plainly medicines fall into the category of products for which the individual consumer cannot adequately assess either quality or performance (in many cases) for himself, and prescribers cannot assess quality, i.e. purity, stability, etc.

The four areas in which government acts to control the manufactured product are concerned with

quality
safety
efficacy

[1] William Hamilton, MD: *Observations on the proportion, utility and administration of the Digitalis Purpurea or Foxglove*: Longman, 1807.

supply, i.e. whether available to the public through any shop, or only through pharmacies, or on a doctor's prescription.

A basic principle of control in the public interest is that no medicine may be sold (or supplied) without prior licensing or registration by government. If there is no licensing system there can be no control.

The fact that some medicines are, by general consent, available only on prescription by a doctor or, where sold directly to the public, available only from a pharmacy, is a formal acknowledgement that the general public are not competent to make some judgements, that drugs cannot be completely safe and that what is appropriate for one sick person may not be appropriate for another.

The beginning of substantial government intervention paralleled the proliferation of synthetic drugs in the early twentieth century when the traditional and familiar pharmacopoeia expanded slowly at first and then, in mid-century, with enormous rapidity; intervention was initially confined to safety aspects, and was developed piecemeal as issues arose, until the thalidomide disaster of 1961 caused governments all over the world to rationalize, formalize and extend their control of medicines in single, though often complicated laws.

Governmental controls developed approximately as follows. Safety came first and restrictions were imposed on supply of 'dangerous drugs', especially drugs of addiction, and it is significant that there was actually a UK Act of Parliament entitled The Dangerous Drugs Act.

Then followed controls on quality in manufacture which were stimulated by the introduction of preparations of substances occurring naturally in the body, e.g. insulin (1922). Insulin, on accurate dose of which the lives of large numbers of diabetics depend, is obtained from the pancreatic gland of animals in crude form; it is purified and then must be accurately standardized (on animals) so that its potency is consistent. Inefficient or incompetent manufacture will cause deaths, and since the consumer is not able to determine for himself whether the preparation he is offered is reliable, he requires protection against defective products; the same applies to antibiotics. Therefore government control is essential in the public interest.

Efficacy at first received less attention. In the first half of this century medicinal therapeutics was relatively uncritical, though in the UK a law was passed forbidding advertising to the public of 'cures' for venereal disease, tuberculosis and epilepsy. Drug therapy was based on the assertions derived from the impressions of physicians.

In mid-century methods of formal therapeutic evaluation, though foreshadowed by isolated individuals in the previous two hundred years, became established, and scientific comparisons of the efficacy of new and old medicines became commonplace. But governments did not act to extend control of medicines to include efficacy as well as safety; there was no public pressure for them to do so.

The most effective pressure that persuades politicians that they should act radically and quickly is a public scandal.

The first comparatively comprehensive drug regulatory law prior to thalidomide was passed in the USA in 1938 following the death of about 107 people due to the use of diethylene glycol (a constituent of antifreezes) as a solvent for a liquid formulation of sulphanilamide for treating common infections. The sulphonamide group of drugs, introduced in 1935, was the first major therapeutic advance against common bacterial infections. In 1937 in the USA tablets and capsules of sulphanilamide (a member of this new group of antibacterial drugs) were marketed by a number of firms including the S.E. Massengill Company of Tennessee. In June 1937 the firm's salesmen reported a demand for the drug in liquid form (easier for children to take, etc.). Some sulphanilamide is relatively insoluble in the usual vehicles for liquid medicines a number of other solvents used in industry were tried. Diethylene glycol was effective in dissolving the drug and an 'elixir' was made of drug, solvent, flavouring and water.

No tests in animals were made to determine the toxicity either of the ingredients separately or of the finished product, or to determine whether the mixture was stable, i.e. whether the drug decomposed in the solvent when stored. The firm's laboratory merely checked the mixture for appearance, flavour and fragrance. No special trials were conducted in man; 240 gallons (1,100 litres) of the mixture were made and marketed. This procedure was compatible with the then existing law in the USA.

In October 1937 news of deaths in Oklahoma was telephoned to the US Food & Drug Administration (FDA) by a physician. Eight children with sore throats and one adult with gonorrhoea had died after taking the 'elixir'. When the Massengill Company heard of the poisonings it sent out 1,100 telegrams to its customers and salesmen asking for collection and return of all 'elixir' that had been sold. Since these requests seemed unlikely to impress receivers with the true urgency of the situation, the investigating FDA inspectors insisted, on 19 October, that a more cogent telegram be sent:

'Imperative you take up immediately all elixir sulphanila-mide you dispensed. Product may be dangerous to life. Return our expense.'

Large amounts were sent back, but it was essential that *all* be recovered. Almost all the 239 FDA inspectors and chemists were assigned to this task. Warnings were broadcast by radio and newspaper. Individual prescriptions were identified and pursued as far as possible, though the pursuit was hampered by prescriptions such as, 'Betty Jane, 9 months old' and 'Mrs Jackson' (no address). But some elixir had been sold directly to the public and the purchasers were unknown.

Massengill Company travelling salesmen were pursued from hotel to hotel and interviewed. One salesman was unco-operative, but changed his mind when jailed. Most doctors and pharmacists co-operated. But one doctor who had admitted dispensing to five patients refused their names though claiming they were all alive. Enquiry revealed he had supplied seven patients and four were dead.

'One of the fatal prescriptions was traced through neighbourhood gossip describing the symptoms of the fatal illness of a Negro employee of a lumber mill. The inspector recognized the symptoms as characteristic of "elixir" poisoning and through the mill superintendent found the victim's sister. She remembered the doctor had given her brother some red medicine about October 2 or 3. She said that in accordance with their custom, all medicines, glasses, spoons, etc., had been placed on the grave, which was about 1½ miles back in the fields. Accompanied by the Negroes, the inspector walked to the wooded knoll with its single mound of fresh earth on which lay several bottles, dishes and spoons. One 4 ounce bottle contained about one ounce of the "elixir". It bore the weatherbeaten but legible prescription label of the doctor.'[2]

Typical effects occurred 24-48 hours after taking the elixir, with nausea, vomiting, malaise, severe abdominal pain and sometimes diarrhoea. Urine production ceased, the patient became unconscious and either died after 2 to 7 days or recovered over 7 to 21 days. Autopsy disclosed damage to the kidneys and liver.

As soon as its help was requested by physicians (11 October 1937) the American Medical Association asked the Massengill Company the composition of the 'elixir' since this was not declared on the label. The Company provided the information, though requesting that it should be treated as confidential.

On 20 October the Company telegraphed the American Medical Association, 'Please wire . . . suggestion for antidote and treatment . . .' and the Association replied, 'Antidote for Elixir Sulfanilamide-Massengill not known . . .'

About 107 people died. The only basis for action under the Food and Drugs Act was that the word 'elixir' traditionally implies an alcoholic solution, whereas this contained diethylene glycol.

On 23 October, Dr Massengill issued a press statement:

'My chemists and I deeply regret the fatal results, but there was no error in manufacture of the product. We have been supplying legitimate professional demand and not once could have foreseen the unlooked-for results. I do not feel that there was any responsibility on our part. The chemical sulfanilamide had been approved for use and had been used in large quantities in other forms, and now its many bad effects are developing.'

The bad effects were in fact due to the diethylene glycol solvent and evidence of possible harm was available prior to marketing this 'elixir'. Effects similar to those in man are easily shown in animals.

[2] Quoted from Report of the Secretary of Agriculture submitted in response to resolutions in the House of Representatives and Senate (USA): *Journal of the American Medical Association* (1937), vol. 109, p. 1985, from which most of this account is obtained.

In November, Dr Massengill stated (in a letter to the American Medical Association), *'I have broken no law.'* In fact a federal court later found that he had broken the law in relation to 'adulteration and misbranding' of an 'elixir' and he was fined $150 on each of 112 counts, making a total of $16,800. But 'Federal officials were miserably handicapped by the weak law'.[3]

Congress now acted quickly and passed a bill providing that no new drug or any modification of old drugs should be placed on the market until the entire formula had been submitted to the Food and Drug Administration of the US Department of Agriculture and the firm licensed to market the drug. Claims made on labels, advertisements, etc., were also brought under supervision of the Federal Trade Commission.[4]

All this took place nine years after a pharmacologist speaking before the Section of Pharmacology and Therapeutics of the American Medical Association (1929) said:

'Many drug firms make the mistake of believing that their chemists can furnish trustworthy pharmacologic opinion. Indeed, some eminent chemists, impatient with careful pharmacologic technic have ventured to estimate for themselves the clinical possibilities of their own synthetics . . . There is no short cut from chemical laboratory to clinic, except one that passes too close to the morgue.'[5]

Other specialists in 1938 listed the technical requirements for developing a drug and commented,

'many more lives will be sacrificed if such standards are not put into effect. Any essential compromise with these requirements will inevitably exact a toll of deaths or injuries among the public. The life and safety of the individual should not be subordinated to the competitive system of drug exploitation.'[6]

[3] *Journal of the American Medical Association* (1938), *111*, 1567.
[4] *Ibid.*
[5] *Ibid.*, 919.
[6] *Ibid.*

Other countries did not learn the lesson provided by the USA and it took the thalidomide disaster of 1960-1 to make governments all over the world initiate comprehensive control over all aspects of drug introduction, prescribing and sale directly to the public. Those governments that already had some control system extended it, but no regulatory system can guarantee complete safety. Therefore it is interesting to consider whether the thalidomide disaster might have been prevented by a routine control system such as that in force in the USA. The USA and the UK have similar attitudes to technical medicine. The former had a comprehensive regulatory body (FDA) in 1960 and the latter did not. It might be thought that this would provide a field test of the usefulness of official drug regulation. But it did not.

Thalidomide was developed in West Germany and introduced thence into other countries. It was marketed in the UK without official review or hindrance but it was delayed in the USA by the routine application of administrative machinery. During this delay period the adverse effect of thalidomide on the nerves to the limbs (peripheral neuritis) was detected during clinical use in the UK. Naturally this led to further cautious delay in the USA and during this further period the harmful effect on the fetus was revealed in other countries.

It is hard to be sure, but it is quite likely that if thalidomide had been first developed in the USA the drug would have been marketed there. There will continue to be speculation, informed by hindsight, whether the substantial freedom of the USA from thalidomide was the result of scientific insight or of bureaucratic caution, or a mixture of the two.

Mere delay protects, provided others are using the drugs concerned. But it can also deprive populations of valuable drugs (see below).

A modern drug regulatory organization requires that scientific evidence be submitted to it of:

1. tests carried out in animals to allow some prediction of potential efficacy and safety in man,
2. chemical and pharmaceutical quality (purity, stability, formulation, etc.),
3. initial limited studies in man (healthy or sick, as appropriate),
4. substantial trials in patients to determine whether the

drug deserves to be licensed or registered for general prescription (the drug being supplied by the developer without charge, for it is not yet a medicine).

But now an extra stage is recognized as necessary: post-registration (marketing) surveillance or monitoring.

Whilst the general ethical aspects of such research programmes are obviously a concern of regulatory bodies, the details are generally a matter for the investigators themselves, advised or supervised by local ethical review committees. Ethics will not be considered further here (see also Chapter 6), not because it is unimportant but because it is part of the wider problem of medical research and needs fuller discussion than can be given here.

But it may be wondered why post-registration surveillance should be necessary. Common sense would seem to dictate that safety and efficacy of a drug should be fully defined before marketing.

Unfortunately this of often not practicable. Pre-registration trials with very close supervision are commonly limited to a hundred or a few hundred patients. Rare serious adverse effects which are unpredicted or unpredictable from studies in animals will either not be seen, or if seen, there may be no way of determining whether they are due to the drug or to independent coincident disease.

Closely supervised pre-marketing trials (particularly where no exciting result is anticipated but merely a possibility of modest advance) constitute a tremendous burden on both the investigator doctors and on patients. Interest of the doctor flags, willingness of patients to accept the inconvenience of close supervision declines, precise records become imprecise, patients drop out. Even if mammoth trials are done (and they are very expensive) there is no certainty of a useful result.

An eight-year study of treatment of diabetes (referred to in Chapter 5) which started in 1961 cost the US Government $7.7 million and has not answered the problems of long-term management of maturity-onset diabetes. Current multi-centre and international studies of drug treatment of mild high blood pressure will take years to complete and already the cost is running into the equivalent of millions of US dollars.

Both the above examples employ drugs already marketed

and shown effective in controlling the blood sugar in diabetics and the blood pressure respectively. But it still has to be proved that close control of blood sugar and of mild high blood pressure is actually accompanied by fewer major complications and longer life. The end result of a long-term treatment over many years can only be discovered by following treated patients over many years. The scale of these studies requires large-scale production of drugs and their use in many thousands of patients. In medical and social terms it seems irrelevant how the drug is being supplied; in any case it must be paid for by somebody, and in fact, ultimately by the public.

Medicines must be allowed to be sold (they are supplied free for clinical trials) at a reasonably early stage if research-based industry is to continue to operate. Of course there will be no question of granting a licence to sell until there is evidence that the majority of patients will benefit. But the rarer risks cannot be accurately determined until as many as 10,000 and even up to 100,000 patients have used the drug. Such experience may take years. The only way in which this experience can be financed is by selling the drug. Selling the drug does not mean its use is not being closely supervised. It is the supervision and evaluation that is important to patients rather than whether it is supplied free or for money. But a flow of money is essential to industry to support manufacture, distribution and research into further new drugs.

The regulatory organization has the power to control the claims and to ensure that necessary information is provided to prescribers and patients so they will not be misled. But allowing sale and general prescribing should no longer mean the end of the period of formal evaluation.

It must be recognized that full evaluation of medicines commonly takes many years. Oral contraceptives, antidiabetic agents and hormone replacement therapy for post-menopausal women are examples where evaluation proceeds over decades. Major tranquillizers are still controversial after more than twenty years of widespread use.

It is evident that where a drug increases the incidence of a disease that occurs spontaneously and commonly, no monitoring system, however efficient, can identify the first drug-induced cases for what they are. For example, the

M.Y.T. – E

increasingly popular use of oestrogens alone (not combined with a progestogen as in oral contraceptives) to relieve the unpleasant menopausal symptoms due to the cessation of natural production of oestrogens and subsequently indefinitely as hormone replacement therapy (HRT) has been shown probably to cause cancer of the lining of the uterus (endometrial cancer) and the incidence increases as therapy is more prolonged (some investigators disagree, stating that these studies are biased).

Such a consequence can only reliably be discovered and confirmed by epidemiological methods and this means large-scale use in women, and certainty grows as more women develop cancer. If this is not acceptable practice then therapy of this kind cannot be introduced at all for the foreseeable future.

Professional medical caution over the possible hazard of HRT has been condemned as an example of the indifference of a male-dominated profession to the suffering of women, and even as a sexist desire (conscious or unconscious) in men to make women suffer. The fact that women doctors expressed equal concern merely shows, it is implied, how successfully men dominate the profession.

The benefits of oestrogens used briefly for menopausal symptoms are not seriously doubted. The benefits used as long-term replacement therapy are controversial. That long-term use of oestrogens reduces post-menopausal thinning of bones, with increased risk of fractures, is possible but that it also increases the incidence of cancer seems probable. It is not merely important to know that this cancer risk is there, but it is essential to know, if at all possible, the magnitude of the effect, because only then can a sensible decision be taken on acceptance or non-acceptance of risk.

It seems that the increased risk is less than that of heavy smoking. In the light of such knowledge the alternatives are to:

1. abandon the use of oestrogens for this purpose (HRT) altogether,
2. use oestrogens in short courses at the lowest effective dose to relieve particularly troublesome symptoms,
3. accept the risk wherever women feel more comfortable taking oestrogen and to prescribe the hormone indefinitely; the woman herself will decide this, for only she

can tell how important are such subjective issues as feelings of well being, possibly postponed facial wrinkling, etc.

In such a situation the function of a drug regulatory body is to ensure that the public and the medical profession are properly informed and to offer advice, prepared in consultation with experts in the field, so that those who do not have the skill, the time or the wish to study the evidence and form their own opinion can yet feel that the best opinion is available to them. It is our opinion that the course suggested in (2) above is the wisest, though we are aware that to some women a wrinkled face is worse than death, and we would not wish to prevent them making their own choice. Hormone replacement therapy is discussed in some detail here, because it exemplifies an increasing trend in our society, the expectation or demand that the natural consequences of ageing, as well as the chronic diseases that are accumulated with age, be relieved or prevented. This objective can only be partially achieved, and it involves continuous administration of hormones, natural or synthetic, as well as of other drugs over very long periods (many years) to increasing numbers. For example, elderly people may find themselves taking post-menopausal hormone replacement therapy, a drug to lower blood lipids to prevent heart attacks, and/or a drug to reduce the sickness of the platelet cells of the blood which are concerned with coagulation, also to prevent heart attacks; in addition they may have high blood pressure and need one or even two drugs for that. If in addition they have rheumatism and bronchitis it will be appreciated how they can quite easily come to be taking five or more different drugs daily for years. It would indeed be a source of surprise rather than the reverse, if such practices did not bring with them problems quite unforeseeable from animal tests or short term use in man. Risks of rare adverse effects which are readily accepted by patients who have had a serious episode of disease are seen in a different light when the drug is used in millions of people in the hope of avoiding disease. A person who has had a serious heart attack has a different view of risk from that of a healthy middle aged person with only slightly raised blood lipids who is invited to take a drug for the rest of his life to prevent something that might in any case never occur. Evaluation of drugs for such preventive purposes presents enormous problems both of medicine and of practicality. Drug regulatory organizations must be concerned with all this.

Though efficacy of a new drug for the intended uses must be shown, safety is the chief driving force behind official drug regulation, as is shown by the name of the UK drug regulatory organization, the Committee on *Safety* of Medicines.

There is an understandable tendency to feel that a substance developed with the objective of relieving suffering should itself be incapable of causing suffering, and that if suffering ensues somebody must be at fault and that he can be discovered and punished. But this feeling is not based on reason, and hazard is as inseparable from introducing chemicals (drugs) into the body as it is from surgery. Everybody knows, indeed it is self-evident, that surgery and anaesthesia (with drugs) carry risks, and most people readily accept them. But the act of prescribing is so brief and seemingly so trivial that it is hard to believe that it can have widespread and even catastrophic effects. It is from irrational feelings that all drug-induced disease is or should be avoidable that there arise public pressures and outcry when things go wrong due to the inevitable inadequacies of drug science.

Those responsible to the public or who might be blamed for an accident, naturally find it hard to resist this pressure. They attempt to meet the essentially unreasonable demand for total safety by increasing the requirements for testing, even where there is no good reason to believe that increased testing gives increased assurance of safety.

For example, before thalidomide it was not a routine practice to test new drugs on pregnant animals. After thalidomide it became the routine to test all new drugs during early pregnancy in animals, at which stage the major organ-forming processes take place. Now testing has expanded to cover risk at all stages of the reproductive process and drugs are administered to male and female animals for weeks before mating, continued in the female throughout pregnancy and until the young are weaned; the young are then reared to reproductive age and their fertility tested by breeding from them.

Thus it is hoped to avoid future accident to any stage of the reproductive process. In fact, little is known of the predictive value of such tests. But there is no doubt whatever as to their cost in money and scientific resources.

Increasingly drugs are tested for carcinogenic effect, for one year in the mouse, two years in the rat and seven years in the dog, and this testing is likely to become a routine requirement (at least in rodents) for all drugs intended for use over long periods in man. Testing for effects on genetic material (mutagenicity) in bacteria and in animals is increasingly being done and is likely to become a routine requirement in the near future. And so it goes on, the labour and cost of drug testing prior to administration to man steadily increases.

This could be justified if there were good assurance that the increase really gave extensive protection to man. But there are grounds for believing that such tests have a limited and uncertain value.

We are not saying that tests in animals are of no use. They are quite essential within their limitations. We would regard the administration to man of chemicals on which there was no information on their effects in animals as quite unacceptable. Biological tests that do not involve animals, e.g. tissue culture, are in their infancy and are not likely ever to become a complete substitute for tests in whole animals. We consider that the pursuit, by public demand and by the natural desire of drug scientists and official regulatory bodies, of virtually absolute safety or 'safety at any cost', even where lip service is sometimes paid to the inevitability of hazard, is now reaching a point where it may, paradoxically, act against the public interest. It may stop the development of new drugs for serious and untreatable disease, especially uncommon diseases, by rendering programmes prohibitively costly.

Already an oral contraceptive must undergo laboratory research and safety testing for ten years (carcinogenicity tests in beagles for 7 years are considered essential) before it can be tried in woman (or man), and there is then no substantial certainty that it will not then fail the necessarily large and rigorous human testing programme.

Whether drugs are developed by private or state enterprise, considlerations of investment of the now enormous resources demanded are liable to turn those responsible to seek other outlets for their skills and for their investment.

We consider that there is a solution.

Put bluntly it is based on the fact that if we want to know for certain if a drug is effective and safe in human disease, it must be put to the test in human disease. In saying this we are not callous, or seeking to transfer the costs of safety testing from the animal laboratory to the clinic. We simply advocate frank recognition of inescapable biological realities and the most efficient use of resources that are both costly and limited.

This means that drugs should undergo a reasonable (in current scientific terms) testing programme in animals. They should then enter a limited period (that will be defined for each drug) of closely supervised testing in man to define provisionally its efficacy and safety.

If the drug is judged to pass these tests successfully then it should be made generally available for prescription, but under special defined conditions (according to whether it is an anaesthetic, an ointment for eczema, an inhalation for asthma, etc.) that will ensure that patients receiving it are individually monitored for unexpected events or for changes in incidence of coincident disease for a period which will often be years. For example, if an adverse effect occurs in 1 in 10,000 (0.01%) patients tested, then to determine this reliably (95% probability) it will be necessary to study at least 30,000 patients. These 'post-registration (marketing) surveillance' techniques are being developed. Such a programme would allow the public to be provided with the new drugs it needs with a minimum of risk.

Risk can be minimized, it cannot be eliminated. Therefore in research and development programmes, which are in the interest of the sick in general as well as of the individual patient, those who accept the risk of the unknown should be appropriately compensated (as far as money and social services can compensate) by the producer or by society if they suffer harm.[7]

Attempts to eliminate risk entirely are unrealistic and will result in depriving the sick of relief. There is good reason to

[7] The issue of responsibility for known adverse effects of drugs accepted for use in routine medical practice presents slightly different problems, see Chapter 3.

assert that this has actually happened in the USA where there has been delay, often amounting to years, in obtaining regulatory approval for useful new drugs for high blood pressure, angina pectoris, infections and asthma.

On the other hand, the USA largely (though not wholly) escaped the accident of thalidomide. It also escaped the accident of practolol (Eraldin), a drug shown to preserve life following myocardial infarction (coronary thrombosis), that causes skin rashes, eye disease sometimes leading to blindness and intestinal obstruction.

It is not easy to quantify benefits that have been missed, but it is relatively easy to quantify damage that has occurred, and it is horror concerning the latter, even when it is on a far smaller scale than motor accidents or accidents in the home, that tends to dominate our attention. Official drug regulation can do a lot of good; that is obvious. It can also do harm, and that is less obvious. The tendency of any government body is to play safe. It is always safer to allow somebody else to take risks rather than to take them oneself.

This is why it is desirable for regulatory decisions to be made on the advice of groups of independent experts (as is the case in the UK) rather than by civil servants whose careers can be at stake (as in the USA, though we understand this may be changing).

Regulatory bodies should also actively encourage drug research and not act solely as policemen as is generally the case at present. Unfortunately, in some countries bad relationships have grown up between drug developers and the regulatory body. There is mutual suspicion and resentment. Industrial drug developers complain of rigid, often meaningless, and so unjustifiable testing requirements as well as of long delays in decision-making that disrupt research programmes.

Regulatory bodies can point to instances of dishonest 'research' and carelessness in industry, and to dishonest reports by doctors who are paid large sums to test drugs and who have occasionally invented results and concealed information unfavourable to the drug.

It is essential that there be mutual confidence and respect between the regulator and the regulated. That these are lacking is due to faults on both sides. The way to rectify this position is as easy to state as it is hard to achieve. All

that is necessary is common sense and good-will with frank-
ness and honesty on the part of drug developers and regulatory bodies. Deliberate dishonesty should be visited with
penalties so severe as to deter even the most amoral scoundrel
from taking risks in this field. The public and politicians
can help by educating themselves and by allowing themselves
to be educated to be reasonable instead of harbouring excessive expectations and fears, and by refraining from
sensationalism and log-rolling when the inevitable accidents
occur; accidents will occur whether or not industry is run
by the state or by private enterprise.

In 1976 the authors participated in a meeting of 17
European drug scientists (of whom four were industrial) on
the Rational Regulation of the Development of New Medicines. The group made a public statement as follows:

'Medicines can never be entirely safe. Despite extensive
testing and monitoring, unforeseen and unpredictable adverse
reactions will continue to occur. The public needs to be
aware that treatment with medicines always carries some risk.
It is the duty of all concerned to maximize benefit and
minimize risk.

'Public concern was deeply aroused by the thalidomide
tragedy and in consequence drug regulatory authorities were
set up or strengthened in many countries. Rules and regulations for drug testing were put forward and, in step with
the laudable intention of increasing safety, the rules have
proliferated. They now place onerous burdens on the manufacturers and investigators of new medicines. There is, however, little evidence that many of the rules do any good or
actually protect the public from harm, while there is much
evidence that they impede innovation.

'There are still fatal and disabling diseases which lack
effective treatment. Mental disorders, arthritis, multiple
sclerosis, psoriasis and many kinds of cancer all await adequate treatment. Resources which could be used for dis-
covering medicines for these diseases are being diverted to
the pursuit of so-called safety, and the public are losing
benefits they might otherwise have.

'The present methods of testing for safety consume time,
money and manpower without a corresponding increase in
safety. Some of them originated soon after the tragedy of

thalidomide and were the most promising which could be devised at the time. They have since been multiplied in the questionable hope that more extensive testing would achieve still greater safety. They have not been altogether successful in achieving their objective. Misfortunes have occurred: the latest, the case of practolol, happened in spite of all the activities of regulatory bodies. Practolol was submitted to and passed every known appropriate test which could be devised by its manufacturer or required by authorities of several nations. It has none the less caused unforeseen injury to hundreds of patients, though this number is a minute fraction of those who have benefited from the drug. In the present state of scientific knowledge, more extensive laboratory testing would not have prevented this misfortune.

'In the opinion of this group of European scientists, it is now advisable to revise our methods of assessment of medicines. We must recognize that existing methods are unsatisfactory. We recommend more rational but less extensive laboratory studies without unnecessary multiplication of detailed clinical trials before registration. Instead we recommend much closer and more extensive surveillance of medicines after they are available for general prescription. Only by the careful study of medicines in everyday use can the greatest benefits be obtained from their administration, the untoward rare potential disaster be recognized at the earliest possible moment, and the ill effects be minimized. Absolute safety is unattainable, and its pursuit regardless of other considerations is achieving more harm than good.'[8]

We believe that it may now be becoming possible for modern society, which has had excessive expectations of science to do nothing but good, to accept that though benefits may be accompanied by risks, sometimes those risks are worth taking.

[8] *European Journal of Clinical Pharmacology* (1977), *11*, 233.

THE THALIDOMIDE DISASTER

This has been a turning point in the history of drug therapy: an account, with commentary, is therefore provided here.

Until 1961 the public took a largely romantic interest in the development and introduction of new drugs and its attention was only turned to the subject when it learned from the press, generally incorrectly, and several times a year, that a major advance or 'breakthrough' had taken place. In 1961 a major breakthrough did occur – man discovered that drug introduction was more hazardous than he had previously believed. The thalidomide disaster aroused public opinion, forced governments to supervise all stages of drug introduction and all concerned with this process got a salutory shock. Our attitude to casual use of drugs can never be, and should never be the same since thalidomide, and therefore the story is given in some detail here.

In 1960-1 in West Germany an outbreak of phocomelia occurred. Phocomelia means 'seal extremities'; it is a congenital deformity in which the long bones of the limbs are defective and substantially normal or rudimentary hands and feet arise on, or nearly on, the trunk, like the flippers of a seal; other abnormalities may occur simultaneously. Phocomelia is ordinarily exceedingly rare.

Most West German clinics had no cases during the 10 years up to 1959. In 1959, in 10 clinics, 17 were seen; in 1960, 126; in 1961, 477. The outbreak seemed confined to West Germany (though a similar but smaller occurrence was simultaneously noted in Australia) and this, with the steady increase, made a virus infection, such as rubella, seem unlikely as a cause. Radioactive fall-out was considered and so were X-ray exposure of the mother, hormones, foods, food preservatives and contraceptives. One doctor, investigating his patients retrospectively with a questionnaire, found that 20% reported taking Contergan in early pregnancy. He questioned the patients again and 50% then admitted taking it; *many said they had thought the drug too obviously innocent to be worth mentioning initially.*

In November 1961 the suggestion that a drug, unnamed, was the cause of the outbreak was publicly made by the same doctor at a paediatric meeting, following a report on 34 cases of phocomelia. 'That night a physician came up to him and said, "Will you tell me confidentially, is the drug Contergan? I ask because we have such a child and my wife took Contergan." ' Several letters followed, asking the same question, and it soon became widely known that thalidomide (Contergan, Distaval, Kevadon, Talimol, Softenon) was probably the cause. It was withdrawn from the West German market in November, and from the British market in December 1961. By that time reports had also come from other countries.

In a series of 46 cases of phocomelia it was found that 41 mothers had certainly taken thalidomide and of 300 mothers with normal babies none had taken thalidomide, between the fourth and ninth week of pregnancy.

Soon more reports were forthcoming and despite the fact that such retrospective studies do not provide conclusive evidence of cause and effect, judgement could no longer be suspended on such an important matter, for the drug was not a vital one. Prospective enquiries were quickly made in ante-natal clinics where women had yet to give birth – though few, they provided evidence incriminating thalidomide. The worst had happened, a trivial new drug was the cause of the most grisly disaster in the short history of modern scientific drug therapy. Many thalidomide babies died, but many live on with grotesquely deformed limbs, eyes, ears, heart and alimentary and urinary tracts.

The West German Health Ministry estimated that thalidomide caused about 10,000 birth deformities in babies, 5,000 of whom survived and 1,600 of whom would eventually need artificial limbs. In Britain there were probably at least 600 live births of malformed children of whom about 400 survived. The world total was probably about 10,000 survivors.

Thalidomide had been marketed in West Germany in 1956 as Contergan, and in Britain in 1958, as Distaval, as a sedative and hypnotic. Its chief merit seemed to be that overdose did not cause coma, probably because, with suitable particle size, elimination balanced absorption; given orally to animals a lethal dose could not be reached. Suicides were disappointed by thalidomide. Liquid formulations introduced later lacked this advantage and serious overdose could occur. Thalidomide seemed a safe and pleasant hypnotic, and no doubt some patients found it preferable to others, but in the context of all drug therapy its advantages were trivial, however worthwhile they may have seemed to victims of insomnia.

Despite the absence of any other notable properties, thalidomide, skilfully promoted and credulously prescribed and taken by the public – it was also sold without prescription – achieved large popularity, it 'became West Germany's baby-sitter'. It was a routine hypnotic in hospitals and was even recommended to help children adapt themselves to a convalescent home atmosphere and was sold mixed with other drugs for symptomatic relief of pain, cough and fever (Grippex, Polygripan, Peracon Expectorans, Valgis, Tensival, Valgraine, Asmaval, etc.). This may help explain the difficulties of patients and of doctors in determining who had had thalidomide and who had not, and the statement, probably true, that some women, knowing the danger of thalidomide from press publicity, but not the confusion that reigns amongst drug names, continued to use their supplies of the drug alone or in a mixture, for none of these prominently featured the non-proprietary name on the label. When a drug is in disfavour the advantages of its non-proprietary name become suddenly obvious to those who promote the use of proprietary names, and so more publicity of its teratogenic effect was under the name, thalidomide, than under the numerous proprietary names.

In 1960-1 it had become evident that prolonged use of thalidomide could cause hypothyroidism and peripheral neuritis. The latter effect was the reason why approval for marketing in the USA, as Kevadon, had been delayed by the US government Food and Drug Administration. Approval had still not been given when the fetal effects were discovered and so general distribution was avoided. None the less some 'thalidomide babies' were born in the USA following indiscriminate pre-marketing clinical trials by 1,270 doctors who gave the drug to 20,771 patients of whom at least 207 were pregnant. Other countries in which cases of thalidomide phocomelia occurred include Australia, Belgium, Brazil, Canada, East Germany, Egypt, Israel, Lebanon, Peru, Spain, Sweden and Switzerland, although the drug was not marketed in all these.

When a drug becomes popular it crosses frontiers. It is

interesting to speculate why modest apparent improvements can give a drug a therapeutic reputation such that people will go to great trouble to get it. Responsibility may perhaps be divided amongst manufacturers who over-promote, doctors who write testimonials on inadequate evidence, thus encouraging over-promotion, the press which so ably both satisfies and stimulates the public appetite for 'wonder-drugs' and the self-deluding vanity of patients that makes them feel it a desired distinction to be able to boast of being under treatment with the latest drug, particularly if it is one which is not available to their associates.

Perhaps the fact that the incidence of phocomelia was greatest amongst children of professional classes reflects the urge of doctors to ensure that their own families, as well as those of their perhaps most demanding or critical patients, should get the very newest and therefore, it is optimistically assumed, the best drugs. Or, as the drug was freely sold in West Germany, it may reflect a greater neurotic desire for self-medication in this group, or merely the ability to pay for it.

So rapidly did the news of the thalidomide disaster spread that some mothers who had taken it knew of the risk weeks before their babies were born. Of course, not all who took thalidomide during the crucial period (37th to 54th days from the first day of the last menstruation) had abnormal babies, perhaps no more than 20%, but there is no reliable figure.

Thalidomide has been a terrible lesson to the world and it deserves to be remembered. Its implications in both human and scientific terms merit the attention of all concerned in medical practice. A few are suggested below:

1. It is impossible to believe that all women in early pregnancy who took or were given thalidomide were in serious need of a sedative or hypnotic and that well-tried drugs had failed to give relief. There was certainly a lot of casual use of 'the latest' drug without good reason. This must never be allowed to happen again. Commercial pressures for widespread use in uncontrolled situations, before a drug is thoroughly tried in controlled situations, though understandable, must be resisted. This may make drugs more expensive but it is undoubtedly the lesser evil.

2. Thalidomide was incriminated a mere 5 years after first marketing, because it was extensively used and because the

abnormalities it caused were both dramatic and unusual. It is not known whether any other drugs in general use are causing fetal loss in early pregnancy or fetal abnormalities of a less obvious kind, e.g. reduction in intelligence; a minor tranquilliser (meprobamate) can cause a reduced 'intelligent quotient' in the young when given to pregnant rats, but the significance, if any, of this for man is obscure. However clinical caution is indicated for 'intelligence is not so freely available that it can lightly be interfered with'.[9]

3. Thalidomide, like other drugs, was not tested on pregnant animals before marketing. All new drugs are now tested thus, but the meaningfulness of the results for man is still uncertain. It is also possible that abnormal babies may result from drugs taken by their fathers.

4. Because prediction of clinical effects from animals is imperfect, machinery for reporting all possible drug toxicity to a central bureau to enable real effects to be detected at the earliest moment is essential and such monitoring schemes have been set up in many countries.

5. Except for demonstrably life-saving introductions, newness of a drug should be regarded as a reason for *not* prescribing it except as part of a scientific evaluation or where older, well-tried drugs have failed, until its place in relation to existing drugs is established.

6. In general, doctors are too ready to prescribe drugs and patients are too ready to take them for conditions which are self-limiting or cause only trivial discomfort.

In 1977 in the UK there were still heard demands for an official public enquiry into the thalidomide disaster.

The present position is that after a long struggle the victims of thalidomide have received a substantial sum of money from the drug firm that marketed thalidomide. It is unlikely that a court of law would have awarded more in the event of the producer being found guilty of negligence, an outcome which remains uncertain.

The medical/scientific lessons provided by the episode have been learned in that an official regulatory body (Committee on Safety of Medicines) has been set up and no new drug is marketed until a body of independent experts has agreed that testing is adequate; claims of efficacy and safety can

9 Editorial (1963), *British Medical Journal, 1*, 138.

also be controlled under law.

The only remaining issues would seem to be:

1. Whether the drug firm was liable *in law* for the consequences of thalidomide. This has not been tested in the courts of law since the firm concerned paid compensation, having admitted 'moral' but not 'legal' liability. The law on 'product liability' ('strict' liability, 'no fault' liability) is currently being reviewed in the UK as well as in many other countries and there seems little point in embarking on what could be an enormous and expensive legal exercise under laws that are about to be changed, partly, indeed, as a result of the thalidomide disaster.

2. Whether anyone has behaved in such a manner that they should be prosecuted for negligence, criminality, concealment of information, etc. We doubt if this is a serious probability in the UK but are not able to comment on the position in other countries.

8. Prescribing and consumption of medicines

1. QUANTITY

Consumption of drugs has become a normal part of daily life in our society. The following supporting data are only a small proportion of what could be quoted.

In the UK on average the 57 million people (patients) consult their doctor three times a year and receive a prescription averaging 1.6 items at two of these consultations. Nearly as many prescription items again are issued without direct contact between doctor and patient.

In a study of prescriptions issued by general practitioners to a population of about 40,000 in the UK[1] in one year it was found that 54% of men and 66% of women had at least one drug dispensed. Psychotropic drugs (affecting behaviour) were prescribed to 10% of males and 21% of females. Of women aged 45-59 years 33% received a psychotropic drug and 11% were given an antidepressant. One psychotropic drug, diazepam (Valium), generally prescribed as a sedative against anxiety and insomnia, was given to 6% of the population.

In an Australian town[2] with 15,700 inhabitants a study of drug use was conducted (in 10% of the households plus 10% of people living in institutions, hotels, etc.). In the two weeks immediately preceding enquiry
only 11% of people reported neither illness nor drug usage;
66% of people had taken some medication;
more than half of these had taken more than one drug;
6% had taken four or more drugs;

[1] Skegg, D. C. G. et al, 1977, *British Medical Journal, 1,* 1561.
[2] Quoted in Wade, D. N. (1976), *Clinical Pharmacology and Therapeutics, 19,* 651.

almost 60% of the medication taken was self-prescribed;
slightly less than 40% was prescribed by a doctor;
2% was prescribed by a pharmacist.

In another study in Melbourne (Australia) it was found
that 30% of the population regularly took drugs.

A survey in nine West European countries[3] disclosed that
the proportion of people using a tranquillizer or sedative
drug was 17% in Belgium and France, 14% in the UK and
10% in Spain. The proportion of women was twice that of
men and use increased with age.

In Eastern Quebec medication, at the time of enquiry, was
being taken by 37% of females and 27% of males, and
regular medication was being taken by 65% of females aged
over 60 years.

In Denmark it has been calculated that every person is
prescribed a dose of tranquillizer every second or third day
and an analgesic every eighth day.

In a study in the UK,[4] in the two weeks prior to enquiry
32% of adults aged over 55 years had taken self-prescribed,
and 52% doctor-prescribed medicines; 44% had taken
some of each. Amongst adults aspirin and other analgesics,
and amongst children skin ointments and antiseptics, were
the most frequently used drugs; the majority of these were
not prescribed by a doctor. One-fifth of the medicines prescribed by doctors acted on the nervous system. It was also
found that 40% of adults took some medicine every day in
the two weeks before enquiry. 75% of these daily medicines
were obtained on repeat prescriptions, and 25% of regular
medicine takers were using medicines prescribed a year or
more ago. 'So, for a sizeable proportion of people, medicine
taking has become a habit often encouraged, or at least
supported by their doctors.'[5]

The Australian study quoted above also lists the nature
of medications taken in an urban community in the following order: analgesics, cough and cold suppressants, vitamins
and tonics, comprising together half the total consumption;
antibiotics are a close fourth followed by drugs for skin

[3] Balter, M. B. et al (1974), *New England Journal of Medicine,*
290, 769.

[4] Dunnell, K., Cartwright, A. (1972), *Medicine Takers, Pre-*
scribers and Hoarders: Routledge & Kegan Paul, London.

[5] *Ibid.*

diseases, diseases of the heart and circulation, hormones, drugs acting on the nervous system (tranquillizers, sedatives), antirheumatic drugs, and antacids (for indigestion).

Consumption of both self and doctor-prescribed drugs has increased rapidly over the past ten years in Australia, the USA and the UK. The author of the Australian study already quoted writes, 'By any standards Australians are near the top of the world "Hit Parade" of drug takers.' It seems that 60% of Australians average two or more doses of analgesics per day. In the UK it is estimated that one night's sleep in ten is drug assisted. In the UK, prescribing by family doctors grows at 5% per annum (in real terms, i.e. allowing for inflation). It is one of the fastest growing sectors of the health and personal social services budget.

It is evident that people have an increasing desire for medicines and that this is well catered for by manufacturers and doctors. The question arises whether this desire is solely the result of a true medical need, i.e. whether the drugs are curing or preventing disease. We do not think it is. We agree with the Australian author who suggests that drug consumption in our societies is unnecessarily high and that it causes a significant burden of drug-induced disease, that current levels of drug use are probably symptomatic of underlying stresses and pressures in urban societies together with a cultural background that accepts the social use of drugs and encourages high expectations in relation to health with a low threshold of what constitutes illness.

In this connection we have heard of two European countries where colleagues have had the experience of being offered with their after-dinner coffee an analgesic and a purgative respectively. We hope that such practices are exceptional, but it is striking that they could happen at all.

2. DOCTORS AND PRESCRIBING

When a patient is given a medicine his responses are the aggregate of a variety of factors:
1. the biological (pharmacodynamic) effect of the drug and its interaction with any other drugs the patient may be taking,
2. the physiological state of the target organ, whether, for

instance, it is over- or underactive,
3. the act of medication, including the route of administration and the presence or absence of the doctor,
4. the doctor's mood, personality, attitudes and beliefs,
5. the patient's mood, personality, attitudes and beliefs,
6. what the doctor has told the patient,
7. the patient's past experience of doctors,
8. the patient's estimate of what he has received and of what ought to happen as a result,
9. the social environment, e.g. whether alone, or in company.

Obviously some of the above items overlap – the patient's beliefs, for example, being determined by what the doctor tells him as well as by information from other sources, and not every item applies in every case.

The relative importance of these factors varies according to the circumstances – an unconscious patient with meningitis may be assumed to respond to penicillin only in so far as it affects the invading bacteria, and regardless of whether he and the doctor dislike each other, but a patient sleepless with anxiety because he cannot cope with his family responsibilities may be affected as much by the interaction of his own personality with that of the doctor as by the hypnotic drug prescribed by the latter; the same applies to appetite suppressants in food addicts.

The physician may consciously, or perhaps more often unconsciously, exploit the factors listed above in his therapeutic practice.

Leo Tolstoy, in 1867, writing[6] of how his heroine's illness, psychosomatic, if not entirely psychological, had been brought on by the vicissitudes of her emotional life, explained how the physical effects of drugs are in some cases irrelevant to the use of medicines. Natasha

'was so ill that [her parents] could not stop to consider how far she was to blame for all that had happened, while she could not eat or sleep, was growing visibly thinner, coughed and, as the doctors gave them to understand, was in danger . . . But it never occurred to one of them to make the simple reflection that the disease Natasha was suffering from could not be known to them, just as no complaint afflicting a living

[6] *War and Peace*, trans. R. Edmonds, Penguin Books, 1957.

being can ever be entirely familiar, for each living being has his own individual peculiarities . . . This simple reflection could not occur to the doctors . . . because medicine was their life-work, because it was for that that they were paid and on that that they had expended the best years of their lives. But the chief reason why this reflection could never enter their heads was because they saw they unquestionably were useful . . . Their help did not depend on making the patient swallow substances, for the most part harmful (the harm was scarcely appreciable because they were administered in such small doses) but they were useful, necessary and indispensable because they satisfied a moral need of the sick girl and those who loved her – and that is why there are and always will be pseudo-healers, wise women and homoeo-pathists. They satisfied the eternal human need for hope of relief, for sympathetic action, which is felt in the presence of suffering, the need that is seen in its most elementary form in the child which must have the bruised place rubbed to make it better . . . The doctors in Natasha's case were of service because they kissed and rubbed the bad place, assuring her that the trouble would soon be over if the coachman drove down to the chemist's in Arbatsky Square and got a powder and some pills in a pretty box for a rouble and twenty kopecks, and if she took those powders in boiled water at intervals of precisely two hours, neither more nor less . . .

'What would Sonya [her sister] have done without the glad consciousness that at first she had not had her clothes off for three nights running, so as to be in readiness to carry out the injunctions promptly, and that she kept awake at night so as not to miss the right time for giving Natasha the not very harmful pills from the little gilt box. Even Natasha herself, though she declared that no medicines could do her any good and that it was all nonsense, found it pleasant to see so many sacrifices being made for her, and that she had to take medicine at certain hours. And it was even pleasant to be able to show, by disregarding the doctor's prescriptions, that she did not believe in medical treatment and did not value her life . . .

'In spite of all the vast number of little pills Natasha swallowed, and all the drops and powders . . . youth prevailed . . . and little by little her health improved.'

But it is still not enough that a patient gets better, it is essential to know *why* she does so. This is because potent drugs should only be given if their biological effects are needed. If other factors are the effective agents, then any drug given will act as a placebo and placebos should at least be harmless.

It is evident that whilst much prescribing for serious disease, e.g. pneumonia, high blood pressure, is based on scientific pharmacology, there is much more to prescribing than science alone. It could be said that prescribing is an art based on science.

In a Scottish study[7] of general practitioner prescribing it was found that no drug was prescribed in 35% of consultations, one drug in 52% and more than one in 13%. Each practitioner used, on average 116 different preparations out of the thousands available. Of all prescriptions 19% were for antibiotics, 9% for cough suppressants and 8% for hypnotics and sedatives.

Patterns of prescribing are known to vary from area to area in a way that is not related to disease pattern. In a study in North Carolina (USA)[8] in which observers watched nearly 100 doctors at work over about 3 days, it was concluded that the less knowledge the doctor obtained in examining a patient, the more drugs he tended to use. In Montreal (Canada) a study showed that, when a physician signed a prescription for a single formulation containing several drugs, in most instances he did not know what the ingredients were and indeed was quite often unaware that the preparation contained more than one drug.[9] The author of the study remarked that if, as the pharmaceutical industry claims, it is an important force in educating doctors about drugs, then either it is a poor educator or the doctors are poor pupils; perhaps both are true.

But this does not alter the fact that doctors have a responsibility to their patients which they cannot be said to be meeting when they do not know what it is they are adminis-

[7] Berkeley, J. S. et al (1973), *Journal of the Royal College of General Practitioners.* 23, 155.

[8] Peterson, O. L. et al (1956), *Journal of Medical Education,* 31, No. 12: pt. 2.

[9] Biron, P. (1973), *Canadian Medical Association Journal, 109,* 35.

tering; if they cannot meet this minimum responsibility they should not prescribe.

The *Journal* of the Royal College of Physicians of London is not an organ that would be expected to be over-ready to criticize the medical profession. In 1976 an editorial stated

'doctors do not employ their critical faculties as they should to every prescription. Indeed the profession as a whole can be criticized for not using the drugs available to the best advantage . . . The only possible conclusion is that a prescription is often born of muddled motives and inadequate knowledge . . .'

One of the troubles is that prescribing is an all-too-easy activity; it requires only a pen and paper. It can be used to terminate an interview with an unhappy patient for whom the doctor can do little or nothing, and doctors are human, they get tired, they get hungry and they are liable to wish to escape from insoluble problems of life, such as other people's unhappiness or incurable sickness.

Putting a chemical into the body can be as hazardous as putting a knife into the body (surgery). Prescribing requires a scribble on a piece of paper and is conducted in relative privacy. Surgery requires extensive facilities and is a relatively public activity carried out before others capable of judging its appropriateness and the skill with which it is performed.

The editorial continues,

'if the doctor had to fetch each bottle of pills and was to find the more dangerous or expensive drugs on the topmost shelf, the effort involved might give his thoughts a rational pause. Some comparable effort might be demanded of the patient. Of course, those who accuse doctors of wantonly scattering pills may be relieved to hear that the number swallowed is only a portion of those scattered. To use the current jargon, prescribing has to be set in the context of patient compliance. That is an odd word, implying that the patient is putty in the doctor's hands. In practice it is not such an unequal contest. Those who demand prescriptions are balanced by those who are suspicious of the best of drugs. Maybe the mass media, which seem intent on spreading the idea that the medical profession is quite ignorant of the drugs it uses, will inculcate among patients a healthy scepticism that will allow them to co-operate more intelligently with their doctors . . .

'The suggestion that anyone would benefit from a law restricting the rights of a doctor to prescribe is so curiously inept that one wonders what sort of bureaucratic or even dictatorial frame of mind would give birth to such an idea.'

The editorial adds that 'the sternest critics [of bad prescribing] are doctors', and this is true.

Recrimination and abuse will not solve the problem which is both large and complex.

There has been an 'explosion', not only of drugs, but of information throughout medicine. It is no longer possible for the individual doctor to have at his fingertips all the knowledge necessary to practice medicine efficiently if he has to cover a wide area of medicine, as is the case with general practitioners.

It may indeed be true, as a past Chairman of the UK Medicines Commission has written, that 'doctors of my generation, particularly those in general practice have no idea how to use, I suppose, 90% of modern drugs'. But it is also true for the authors of this book, specialists in drugs, that when we or our families are taken ill, we send for help to our general practitioners, for these are doctors of broad knowledge and experience who hold the front line in coping with sickness in the community and they are not to be condemned because their technical standards are not those of specialists in each of a multitude of areas of medical management. But despite this, there is not only room for improvement in knowledge and utilization of drugs by both doctors and public, there is also justification for real concern about attitudes to drugs and sense of responsibility within and without the medical profession. If the medical profession and the pharmaceutical industry do not put their houses in order they must expect that public demand will activate the politicians to do it for them in areas both of safety and of economy.

Maybe it is impracticable usefully to legislate to improve prescribing. But politicians anxious to please the electorate as well as to make the world a better place are willing and able to try.

The most recent attempt to restrict medical prescribing rights in the UK was the introduction by a Member of Parliament in 1976 of a short private Bill 'to restrict the right of medical practitioners to prescribe drugs unless certain conditions have been met'.

The Member (Labour Party), seeking leave to introduce the Bill acknowledged that

'there have been many benefits to society from new and powerful drugs developed in recent years, but there has been increasing concern at the adverse effects associated with many of these drugs and at the increasingly casual way in which they are sometimes prescribed by doctors.'

He gave some statistics on prescribing and then said: [10]

'Are we in such a situation that people need that level of prescription – indeed, the almost routine, mindless prescription – of drugs many of which have adverse effects?

'We know that almost 3 per cent of all admissions to hospital are due to adverse drug reactions, and we also know that another 2 per cent or more of admissions to hospital can be traced to drug overdosage. However, even those figures probably understate the problem. We have yet to discover the proportion of patients who recover, not from the effects of any drug which they have been prescribed but simply because those drugs are taken away from them once they have been admitted to hospital. In addition, 10 to 15 per cent of patients develop adverse reactions to drugs during their stay in hospital . . .

'Those effects are avoidable if doctors are made fully aware of the problems. I do not want to overdramatize the situation, but I should like to mention the case of one of my constituents who for over 10 years was prescribed one of the most potent steroids. She developed gross muscle-wasting and weakness, skin atrophy of such a severity that sheets of skin sheared off with a stroke of the hand, and severe bone atrophy resulting in a fractured thigh bone which required a surgical pinning operation for its repair. The patient also suffered high blood pressure and diabetes, and there were no therapeutic benefits whatever in respect of the arthritis from

[10] *Hansard*, 5 May 1976.

which she was suffering.

'There is increasing concern at the cost of drugs and at the waste of many drugs. I believe that Parliament should take steps to control this area of public spending. Perhaps I could offer one further statistic to the House. It is now more expensive to pay for a general practitioner's drug prescriptions than it is to pay the general practitioner his salary . . .

'In this area of activity, public education is important. My Bill aims to increase the level of education among the medical profession itself because I believe that that is an important consideration which is often forgotten. After all, it is the doctors who are supposed to know about these matters and who, in turn, should safeguard the public.

'I should like to see doctors undertaking more drug related education. In recent years there has been a greater development of the specialism of clinical pharmacology . . .

'My Bill aims to capitalize on that expertise by making it more readily available, in particular to general practitioners but also to medical practitioners in the round. My Bill would restrict the prescribing of medicines by fully registered medical practitioners to a small list of relatively safe, innocuous substances drawn up by the Medicines Commission. The medical practitioners would be restricted to providing those drugs, and those drugs only, unless they fulfilled certain criteria.

'The two main criteria are these. First, medical practitioners should attend a minimum of four full (educational) sessions a year on drug-related topics . . . as approved by a postgraduate dean. Secondly, they should make their patients' records available for scrutiny by professional medical audit panels appointed by the regional boards so that any dangerous trends in their prescribing practices could be picked up and discussed with their professional colleagues.

'I do not want to go into the routine detail which is set out in the Bill, but if we were to insist that, in addition to the 10 (educational) sessions that medical practitioners currently have to do to qualify for seniority payments, they should also attend four additional sessions on drug-related topics substantial benefits could be derived . . .

'In addition to this educational provision, the Bill contains one further major provision. It provides that no doctor may prescribe for any patient whom he or his partners have not seen for three months previous to the writing of the prescription. The repeat prescription game is in danger of getting substantially out of hand. There are patients who receive the same medication month in, month out, year in, year out. Without ever seeing a doctor. That sometimes suits the patients and it sometimes suits the doctor.

'I have heard it said, although I have no concrete evidence of it, that some doctors even pre-sign their prescription forms and allow the receptionist to fill out the prescriptions . . .

'I know that there will be concern in the medical profession about my proposals. The profession has already looked at itself in a number of these areas. Last year the BMA [British Medical Association] conference debated the question of the use of barbiturates but, against the wish of its executive came down against any form of voluntary ban on the prescribing of barbiturates.

'I am not proposing any bureaucratic interference in the rights of doctors to treat their patients as they think best, but the doctors will be criticized if they do not develop further educational provision. The audit which I have suggested would be carried out not by civil servants but by professional colleagues.

'It is Parliament's duty to stop what is in danger of becoming a national scandal, and I hope that the medical profession will realize that unless a halt is called soon in this area the profession itself will be damaged by the developments that result.'

Another Member (Conservative Party), replying, said:

'I was concerned when I saw . . . a proposal to restrict the right of medical practitioners to prescribe drugs. I ask the House to think carefully and to reject the proposal . . . With respect to him [the proposer] it sounds like another piece of dogmatic, theoretic, Socialist nonsense.

'I do not dispute that too many drugs are being prescribed in this way. But that has more to do with the level of prescription charges than anything else, and the thought of audit panels being set up fills me with alarm. The hon. Gentleman referred to a small list of relatively safe drugs. What he proposes is a dangerous practice which would put even more power into the hands of the administrators . . .

'The idea of setting up audit panels to scrutinize patients' needs smacks of *1984*. We already have from the Government State-only health proposals. If the hon. Gentleman's proposal were to see the light of day we should end up with State-only prescriptions. I suppose the next step is State-only illness and a person will not be allowed to be ill unless he is suffering from an illness laid down by a panel and agreed to be a proper illness . . .

'My understanding of the position is that no two doctors use the same medicine in exactly the same way and that they find from experience which medicines produce the best results in their hands. Any attempt to restrict the doctor in his choice of medicines would prevent the individual practitioner from using his optimum therapy, which would not be in the interests of patients.

'[The proposer] produced no evidence that he was asking to introduce the Bill specifically at the request of a responsible body of the medical profession. The medical profession has taken a sufficient bashing in the past two years without having its freedom further restricted in this way. Doctors are finding that their skills are not being rewarded financially and they are emigrating. Doctors are disgruntled about the Government's attitude over pay-beds.

'However well intentioned the Bill may be, it is nevertheless a bad Bill. The road to hell is paved with good intentions . . .

'Whilst not doubting the hon. Gentleman's motives, I appeal to the House to take no action until more evidence is produced that this is what the medical profession wants. I ask the House not to give the hon. Gentleman leave to bring in a Bill which would remove from doctors the freedom to practise medicine to the best of their ability.'

These quotations well illustrate the somewhat oversimple attitudes of politicians to this topic, e.g. that adverse reactions to drugs can be avoided by giving information, and that this can be legislated for (information helps, of course).

Commenting on the Bill, the *Lancet*[11] stated that it stood no chance of becoming law and that it was

[11] *Lancet* (1976), *1*, 1249.

'purely a propaganda exercise designed once again to bring attention to the concern about the amount of drugs being prescribed. Although the legislation may be contentious, the concern which lies behind it is now shared widely by Members of Parliament of all parties.'

It added that the major issue was clinical freedom, and this was an area where governments trod softly. If education of doctors in prescribing failed to improve the situation 'then Bills like [this] may become more than just propaganda exercises'. Later the *Lancet* added

'the real issue, of course, is whether a doctor really has the right to prescribe what he likes to whom he likes for as long as he likes. We can hardly criticize civil servants for overspending when the right to prescribe is demanded without acceptance of the responsibilities which go with it.'[12]

Whilst some of the above account is applicable only in societies where the State pays most of the drug bill it seems likely that the problem will become of increasing relevance in societies where, if only for the present, private practice is the principal form. If the State cannot easily pay the bill, then insurance agencies and individuals are likely soon to find the same difficulty.

Legislation in such an area is as liable to create problems as to solve them. With an informed and sensible public and medical profession there should be no need even to think of such legislation on prescribing.

Whilst some of the figures given by the proposer of the Bill (above) might be questioned in detail, many doctors will recognize that there is enough truth in the general account to make them blush.

Some doctors seek to dismiss this kind of critical statement because they can prove an inaccuracy here or there. This is a mistaken and unwise attitude. Somehow the public and its representatives have acquired an anxiety about the way drugs are used and their cost. This anxiety is widespread and is not confined to a disaffected antiprofessional minority, although such people are some of the most vocal in the chorus of concern.

The position is that drug prescribing involves technical knowledge and wisdom as well as social pressures. There is no easy solution to the problems in simply providing more widespread technical education, important though that is. Attitudes must be changed.

Doctors overprescribe. But the public demands medicines for its ills and unhappinesses and commonly puts great pressure on doctors who seek to limit their prescribing to those who actually are likely to benefit from a particular drug (see below on repeat prescriptions). No doubt doctors should resist such pressures, but these are often insistent, and doctors are not exempt from ordinary human feelings, especially when overworked; in many countries the average consultation time is less than five minutes per patient.

The public is concerned both about adverse effects of drugs and cost. It is always convenient to blame someone else for one's shared follies. Doctors are at fault but so are the public. Doctors who should know about medicines have a responsibility to educate the public as well as themselves, but the public must also be willing to be educated and to accept that a prescription is not a necessary culmination of a consultation. Prescription of drugs to mitigate distress where the illness or unhappiness has a primarily social cause that cannot be removed is sometimes necessary in individual cases, but in general it encourages the belief that drugs can do what they cannot do and it distracts from true remedies, namely to change one's way of life, one's environment and society, difficult though such changes always are.

3. PATIENTS AND PRESCRIBED DRUGS

It might be assumed that once a patient has been given a prescription by a doctor he will obtain the drug and actually consume it. The assumption would be wrong, for example approximately 7% of prescriptions issued in an English mining community[13] were never presented for dispensing. Where patients have to pay the full cost of a prescription

[13] Waters, W. H. R. et al (1976), *British Medical Journal, 1,* 1062.

this can have a simple economic explanation. But in this case the prescription charge in the National Health Service was modest and it was men aged 25-34 years who were least likely to present the prescription, whereas in the same community those of children and the old were nearly always presented. The reason suggested in this study was that these relatively young men had to go to the doctor for a sickness certificate to claim National Insurance pay when unable to work, and that they considered the medical content of the consultation as irrelevant and rejected the offered medication. In other communities the rate of non-presentation of prescriptions has been estimated as 1% to 5%.

Further, having obtained the medicine, some 3% to 50% of patients do not take it at all, or if they do take it, do not accurately follow the prescriber's instructions; in depressed out-patients the rate of non-compliance (or non-adherence) can be as high as 70%.

Factors promoting non-compliance include the patient's personality and education level, social isolation, the kind of medicine, the number of medicines being taken concurrently, frequency of administration, duration of treatment, whether the patient feels ill (e.g. acute bronchitis) or quite well (e.g. moderate high blood pressure).

The patient's relationship with his doctor is also important. It has been found that if he feels satisfied with his consultation and the interview was conducted in a friendly rather than in a businesslike fashion, then he or she (there is no sex difference here) is more likely to comply with prescribing instructions. Unfortunately in more than half of doctor-patient consultations the patient does not overtly state his expectations, so that patient satisfaction will be highly dependent on the intuition, willingness to take time and even on the mood of the doctor as well as on the interaction of his personality with that of the patient. Everyone knows that some patients dislike some or all doctors; it is also the case that some doctors dislike some, let us hope not all, patients; no doubt this should not be so, but it is.

Simple failure of comprehension and memory are also obviously important in complying with instructions and these are not helped by a general absence, in most patients, of even the most elementary concept of how the body works and of disease; 'thus approximately 50% of a lay population will not be able to point to the general area of the kidneys, heart, stomach or lungs when presented with outline drawings of the body'. This is demonstrated from time to time on television shows and much laughter is generated by the grotesque concepts of anatomy revealed.

'Patients often have active misconceptions. Only about 10% of patients with peptic ulcer have a reasonably clear idea that acid is secreted by the stomach. Many think that it comes from the teeth when food is chewed, or from the brain when food is swallowed.'

'Another [misconception] is that medication can be discontinued as soon as the patient starts to feel better, a situation commonly seen when antibiotics have been prescribed.'[14]

In one study of sore throat in children treated at home, penicillin by mouth was prescribed for ten days. By the third day over half the children were no longer receiving the drug and by the sixth day nearly three-quarters had ceased to take it. It has been estimated that one-third of prescribed antibiotics are never taken.

Patients also are often diffident about asking nurses and doctors for explanations or repetitions when they are not clear or have forgotten. This is particularly important at first consultations when the patient may be told his diagnosis for the first time and it applies even where the patient shows no overt anxiety.

Clear and repeated instructions using short words and supplemented by written matter (especially for the old) can greatly improve compliance, as can engaging the patient as an understanding participant in the management of his disease, e.g. high blood pressure, rather than as a simple recipient who is subject only to exhortation to do as he is told with threats of displeasure or disaster if he does not.

Studies of what patients remember of what the doctor has told them give results that will occasion no surprise. About one-third of patients have been found unable to recount instructions immediately on leaving the doctor's consulting room; brevity, clarity and repetition by the doctor

[14] Ley, P. (1977), *Prescribers' Journal*, 17, 15.

improve patient recall. Proper labelling of the container supplied to the patient naturally also helps.

A remarkable instance of non-compliance with hoarding was that of a 71-year-old man who attempted suicide and was found to have in his home 46 bottles containing 10,685 tablets. Analysis of his prescriptions showed that over a period of 17 months he had been expected to take 27 tablets of several different kinds daily.[15]

A curious by-way of medicine has been uncovered in investigations of patients who are having 'repeat prescriptions' from their doctors. About two-thirds of general practice prescriptions are for repeat medication (half issued by the doctor at a consultation and half via the receptionist);

95% of patients' requests are acceded to without further discussion,

25% of patients who receive repeat prescriptions have had 40 or more repeats,

55% of patients aged over 75 years are on repeat medication. In a survey[16] of over 50,000 patients of 20 general practitioners it was revealed that:

2.8% of patients had been receiving a daily dose of a psychotropic drug (e.g. tranquillizer, sedative) for at least one year.

The average time since starting this was 5.2 years.

80% of these long-term consumers were aged over 40 years.

75% of them were women.

The numbers of these patients had increased by 80% in 10 years.

Of 31 patients taking a psychotropic drug in 1957, 24 were still doing so in 1967.

Any suspicion aroused by the above facts that prescriptions are desired by the patients and provided by the doctors for reasons unrelated to the biological effects of the drugs is confirmed by analysis of patients who received the same preparation for above 6 months, and often for years – 'long-repeat patients'. These people, it was concluded, are unhappy, and their unhappiness manifests itself as unpleasant bodily

[15] Smith, S. E. et al (1974), *Lancet, 1*, 937.

[16] Balint, M. et al (1970), *Treatment or diagnosis: a study of repeat prescriptions in general practice*. Tavistock, Lippincott.

sensations. The doctor can find no definite disease, but he goes on trying and makes multiple diagnoses, often psychiatric. However, since no satisfactory diagnosis is established, no rational therapy can be provided. The patient continues to complain and the doctor continues to try unsuccessfully. Eventually doctor and patient take refuge uneasily in 'long-repeat prescriptions'. Of course, a proportion of patients taking the same drug for years are doing so for the best reasons, i.e. firm diagnosis for which rational therapy is available, e.g. epilepsy, diabetes, high blood pressure.

4. DRUGS IN THE HOME

In the UK a survey[17] has shown that 99% of the homes investigated contained one or more medicines. The average number of items was 10.3 (3 prescribed, 7.3 non-prescribed); nearly all had some kind of analgesic and skin cream; onefifth had sedatives, tranquillizers or sleeping tablets and twofifths had one or more items that the informant could not identify. In only two of 686 homes were any medicines locked up; medicines were most commonly kept in the kitchen.

From time to time there are campaigns to collect all unwanted drugs from homes in an area. Usually the public are asked to deliver the drugs to their local pharmacies.

In one UK city of 600,000 population, 500,000 'solid dose units' (tablets, capsules, etc.) were handed in. In another of about one million population about one million solid dose units were recovered. Liquid preparations were not accurately measured but over 100 gallons (450 litres) were returned. The total cost of the medicines handed in was estimated (1977 values) at about £28,000 (US $45,000). The organizers of the second study thought the amounts would have been larger if there had been better organization.

One collection comprised the following (dose units or containers) from about 500 households: [18]

[17] Dunnel, K., Cartwright, A. (1972), *Medicine Takers, Prescribers and Hoarders*. Routledge & Kegan Paul.
[18] Nicholson, W. A. (1967), *British Medical Journal*, 3, 730.

Tablets & capsules	43,554
ampoules	194
bottles of medicine	83
liniments	16
ointments & lotions	56
eye drops & ointments	17
ear drops	13
nose drops	17
lozenges	131
powders & cachets	123
pessaries & suppositories	178
miscellaneous	46

It should be remembered that these are preparations that are unwanted in the sense that the owners no longer feel any need to keep them; they are not the whole medicine store of the households.

It is desirable that there be home-prescribing or self-prescribing wherever medicines may be made available without unacceptable risk. The decision as to what risk is unacceptable should be made by level-headed members of the public in consultation with doctors. The fact that some accidents will happen and some abuses will occur is not a reason for refusing to consider enlarging the range of home remedies. Whether aspirin would, if it were now discovered, be considered suitable for general sale is certainly debatable; but despite the deaths and illness aspirin causes, no one now seriously advocates restricting it to a doctor's prescription only. It was undoubtedly right initially to restrict oral contraceptives to doctor's prescription, but now that so much is known about them many reasonable people experienced in the area consider that prescription could safely be widened to other health workers given brief special training, though not at present to direct supply to the public for self-prescription.

But antibiotics should remain available only on a doctor's prescription, for indiscriminate use promotes the spread of drug-resistant bacteria so that infections become untreatable or treatable only with the less safe drugs. In addition some particularly serious bacterial infections, e.g. of the heart valves, are partially suppressed by casual use or wrong choice of antibiotic, so that accurate diagnosis is prevented or delayed until fatal damage has been done by the smouldering infection.

Medicines for self-medication should generally be confined to symptoms where accurate diagnosis of cause is not required, for short-term relief of a symptom and where the margin of safety of the drugs used is substantial.

5. THE PHARMACIST[19]

In the UK medicines are available in three ways, on a doctor's prescription only, by direct sale to the public from a pharmacy only, and by direct sale to the public from any retail outlet. The role of the retail pharmacist has changed a lot with the development of modern manufacturing industry. No longer does he actually make or formulate the majority of prescriptions himself. Yet the pharmacist carries considerable responsibility both in relation to prescribed medicines and to direct sale and advice to the public. The pharmacist has had an extensive training. His skills and potential are currently undervalued and underused in our health system. In the UK the number of local pharmacies is declining under economic pressure. The public may come to regret the loss of this national network of people trained to provide advice and supervision of the use of medicines in the community.

6. COST OF PRESCRIBED DRUGS

The UK National Health Service currently consumes about 6% of the Gross National Product (about 4% in 1951). Pharmaceutical services (medicines, pharmacists, dispensers, etc.) have comprised 8-10% of the total annual National Health Service expenditure over the past 25 years.

Between 1949 and 1975 the number of family doctor written prescriptions rose by 55% and the total cost of prescriptions increased by thirteen times.

[19] Pharmacy traditionally comprises the preparation and dispensing of medicines.

9. The role of industry

Whether drugs are wholly synthetic (made from relatively simple chemicals), semi-synthetic (modifications of complex natural substances) or wholly obtained from natural sources (animal e.g. insulin, plant e.g. digoxin, mould e.g. penicillin or bacteria e.g. asparaginase) they all are the products of a sophisticated chemical industry.

First the pure chemical drug substance is made to statutorily controlled, and very high, standards of chemical purity. Having made the drug it then has to be put into a form that can be taken easily, and travel to and be stored in any climate for long periods without deterioration; these are no small requirements and organizations that can meet them have cause for satisfaction and pride.

The product must be nigh perfect when it leaves its manufacturer; governmental controls are increasingly strict and regulatory authorities are increasingly unsympathetic to those who fall below these standards. In many countries drug manufacture is permitted only in registered and regularly inspected premises.

Formulation of a drug into a medicine is a highly technical procedure. For example there have been instances where tablets undoubtedly contained the correct amount of drug, but it was not released for absorption in the intestine; errors of this kind can be serious in diseases such as epilepsy where the patient's safety depends on his absorbing exactly the right amount of drug into his body. In one instance involving digoxin tablets a change in the tablet-making machinery reduced the amount of drug available to the patient from 80% of the dose swallowed to only 20%; even the pressure to which the formulated drug is exposed during compression in the tablet-making machine can seriously alter its 'bioavailability'.

In most industrialized countries drug research and manufacturing is in the hands of private industry operating in a relatively free market economy. Therefore the drugs made must be priced. Although only industrialists really know how this is done it seems reasonable to suppose that in addition to actual costs of raw materials, manufacture, overheads, and ongoing research,[1] firms must also allow for the costs of patents, obsolescence of their drugs, product competition from, and new discoveries by, other firms and the costs of marketing.

If a product is to be marketed it must have a name. Each drug has at least three names, the chemical name (which is usually far too complicated for ordinary use), the non-proprietary drug name and the proprietary registered trade name of the firm (which applies to its own particular formulation): for example one antidepressant is known as –

chemical name – 3-3 (3-dimethylaminopropylidene) – 1, 2: 4, 5 dibenzocyclohepta-1, 4-diene

official/non-proprietary name – amitriptyline

trade names – Laroxyl, Lentizol, Saroten, Triptyzol

It is a standard complaint against the drug industry that its policy of producing new names for the same drug, made often by many different firms or purchased under cross-licensing agreements, confuses therapeutics. The drug firms vigorously defend their policy, but we have never heard a convincing reply to the long-standing contention that there should be one simple official name for each drug and that, where it is important to obtain the product of a particular manufacturer (a minority of prescriptions) the prescriber should write the official name and add after it the initials or name of the firm, e.g. amitriptyline (Roche) or (Warner) or (MSD). The industry is in no doubt about the marketing advantages of the use of trade marks; the medical profession is in no doubt about the advantages of having a single simple name for each drug. There seems to be room for negotiating about this again in the future.

Along with the name must go sufficient technical information to allow the patients who may benefit to be defined and the drug used properly and the physician alerted to potential dangers. The law requires that each medicine actually being promoted must have an official data sheet

[1] In 1976 it was estimated that the cost of developing a novel drug was US $55 million.

giving this information.

But in the market economy in which they operate the law also allows manufacturers to use standard commercial advertising techniques including the press, direct mailings, gifts, magazines which include non-medical articles, e.g. on cars, holidays, investments, subsidized meetings to encourage prescribing and office visits by trained representatives. Much useful information is given, but even a casual acquaintance with some of this material justifies the criticism that there is over-promotion.

An equally casual acquaintance with the medical profession's willingness to be seduced gives substance to some of the pharmaceutical industry's replies to criticisms of its promotional activities. In addition to activities that invite criticism industry sponsors valuable scientific meetings and gives money to research that is not necessarily immediately profitable to itself.

It is not our intention to indulge in cheap criticism of expensive advertising,[2] though here again we are convinced about the need for more calm discussion and negotiation between the producers and consumers. We know that although tempers become hot and doctrinaire positions are defended to the last glass of whisky, those who work for industry are no more all wicked than the consumers, prescribers and regulatory civil servants are all virtuous. Industry comprises a large number of serious scientists and technicians – about half the members of the British Pharmacological Society (a serious scientific society) work in industry – as well as business and sales staff, many of whom are as concerned to live in a just and healthy society as any other large and miscellaneous occupational group.

This book has been written to help people who want to know what drugs are about and where they come from to make for themselves informed opinions such as can only be helpful in solving the undoubtedly important and difficult problems of retaining the socially valuable dynamic exploring capacities of industrial research and development whilst preventing excess and abuse. Society has now taken to itself

[2] In the UK industry spends about 14% of the product of its home sales on promotion. Government proposes that this should be reduced to 10% (*Lancet* (1976), *1*, 817).

statutory control over all aspects of medicines production and use. Let us hope that those powers will be used prudently to correct the numerous problems discussed in this book, and that overenthusiastic desire to reach, via legislation and bureaucracy, a Utopia where we shall all be happy and healthy will not lead to killing a goose that has laid so many golden eggs.

Conclusions

We hope that readers who have come so far with us will agree that:

1. drugs relieve untold suffering and preserve life,
2. drugs can cause unavoidable illness,
3. by rational attitudes to drug use the benefits can be maximized, and adverse effects reduced though not eliminated,
4. a blind faith in 'wonder drugs' is as foolish as a blind rejection of drugs as unnatural and wholly harmful,
5. the medical profession is under justified criticism for uncritical and casual use of drugs,
6. the public, or at least a vocal section of the public, is reluctant to accept that risks are inevitable, and has unduly high expectations of drugs,
7. the public has yet to recognize that it has a substantial part to play and a responsibility to use drugs rationally,
8. blaming the medical profession for not forcing rational drug policies on the public may satisfy the emotions of the public but is unlikely to be successful in improving matters,
9. the drug industry has produced valuable new drugs, as in 1 above, and is adapted to this function,
10. the drug industry though providing much useful information about its products is also prone to excesses in promotion and to the multiplication of similar drugs to an unnecessary degree,
11. the problems of ensuring that patients who will benefit from drugs receive drugs and that patients who will not benefit from drugs do not receive drugs are extremely complex,
12. government drug regulatory authorities, which in their present form derive from justified concern at the thalidomide disaster, can do harm as well as good; that if the public demands benefits but is unwilling to accept any

risks, then the natural bureaucratic reaction will be to eliminate risks at all costs, even though this must mean eliminating at the same time progress in the treatment of disease,

13. these problems will only be solved by addressing ourselves, that is patients, doctors, industry, drug regulatory organizations, politicians to them with a will to solve them by reason and not by blaming everyone except ourselves,

14. the objective, rational drug use, will be assisted by informing the public of the issues so that it can judge for itself, and

Finally, we wish at the end of this book to appeal to the public not to leave the issues we have raised here solely to doctors, scientists, politicians, bureaucrats and the communications media. These all have their own special interests and objectives, and, well-intentioned as they may often be, they cannot be relied on to meet the best interests of that important minority of the population that we all join at some time in our lives, the sick.

Glossary

This glossary includes virtually all the technical terms used in the book whether or not they have been defined in the text.

ACETONE: a ketone that accumulates in the body when metabolism is deranged by lack of insulin in diabetes.

ACETYLCHOLINE: the substance released at nerve endings that passes an impulse on to another cell, e.g. nerve, muscle or gland.

ADRENAL GLAND: lies above the kidney: consists of (a) cortex that produces steroid hormones (chiefly cortisol) that exert widespread control of numerous tissue functions and that are essential to life: and (b) medulla that secretes adrenaline into the blood, plays a relatively minor part in responses to stress and is not essential to life.

ADRENALINE: a substance derived from noradrenaline having similar functions: chiefly produced in adrenal medulla: the word is consistently misspelled by journalists; without the final 'e' it is a proprietary name owned by a drug firm.

ADRENOCEPTORS: the tissue receptors that respond to the hormones noradrenaline and adrenaline and to synthetic adrenaline-like (sympathomimetic) drugs: the adrenoceptors are of two kinds alpha and beta and these can be selectively blocked (by alpha- and beta-adrenoceptor blockers) which are useful in cardiovascular diseases.

ADRENOCORTICAL STEROIDS: natural and synthetic substances related to cortisol (hydrocortisone) the principal natural hormone of the cortex of the adrenal gland: availability in medicine (since 1948) marked a major advance in management of a wide range of immunological and inflammatory disease as well as remedy of deficiency states.

AEROSOL: fine particles dispersed in a gas, either of liquid (fog) or of solid (smoke).

AGRANULOCYTOSIS: a lack of one of the main types of white blood cell (granulocytes) important for resistance to infection: it can occur as a result of allergy to some drugs: it is a serious disease.

ALLERGY: response of the body to a foreign substance (antigen) which induces formation of reactive antibody so that subsequent contact with antigen causes disease, e.g. hay-fever is a pollen allergy.

ALLOPURINOL (ZYLORIC): a drug that blocks an enzyme (xanthine oxidase) that synthesizes uric acid in the body thus lowering the amount of uric acid made: useful in preventing gout.

ALPHA (α) – ADRENOCEPTORS: ALPHA-ADRENOCEPTOR BLOCKING DRUGS: see adrenoceptors.

AMINO ACID: the structural sub-units of proteins.

AMPICILLIN (PENBRITIN): a semi-synthetic penicillin active against a wider range of organisms than the original natural penicillin: but it is somewhat less efficacious, so it does not render its parent obsolete.

AMPOULE: a glass container to hold sterile drug usually for injection.

ANAESTHESIA: after the demonstration by William Morton (USA) that the volatile liquid, ether, could be used to induce unconsciousness and allow leisurely, and therefore better, surgery Oliver Wendell Holmes wrote to him: 'The state should, I think, be called "Anaesthesia". The adjective will be "Anaesthetic".'

ANALGESIC: pain relieving: analgesic drugs may be classified as narcotic (originating from or chemically related to the active principles of opium), e.g. morphine, or non-narcotic, e.g. aspirin: in general the narcotic analgesics are required for severe pain which is beyond the reach of the non-narcotic analgesics.

ANAPHYLACTIC SHOCK: an immunological phenomenon in which the antigen-antibody combination damages cells which release stored histamine which causes collapse of the circulation and bronchial constriction (asthma): severe cases are extremely dramatic: emergency treatment by injected adrenaline and antihistamine: occasionally caused by drugs.

ANDROSTERONE: a male sex hormone.

ANGINA PECTORIS: insufficient blood flow to the heart muscle results in insufficient oxygen delivery and so to pain, especially on exercise.

ANTACIDS: substances that neutralize acid: the principal ingredients of indigestion powders.

ANTIBIOTIC: substance produced by micro-organism that, in high dilution,* is antagonistic to growth or life of other micro-organisms. (*This proviso is necessary to exclude alcohol and hydrogen peroxide which are made by living organisms and which are classed as antiseptics, which see.)

ANTICOAGULANT: drug that reduces capacity of blood to clot: used to treat thrombosis.

ANTIGEN/ANTIBODY REACTION: an antigen is a substance that causes the body to produce substances that combine with it to neutralize it: the combination of antigen with antibody can lead to release from cells of active substances, e.g. histamine, causing symptoms of varying severity: see anaphylactic shock.

ANTIHISTAMINE: a drug that competes with histamine for histamine receptors: being relatively inert it thus prevents histamine from producing its characteristic inflammatory effects.

ANTIHYPERTENSIVE: blood pressure lowering.

ANTIMICROBIAL DRUG: kills or immobilizes microbes, i.e. bacteria, protozoa, etc.

ANTIPYRETIC: reduces fever.

ANTISEPTIC: substance that kills or stops growth of bacteria: usually only applied to substances unsuitable for internal use as medicines.

APLASTIC ANAEMIA: a failure of the bone marrow to make all the cellular elements of blood, red cells (oxygen carrying), white cells (protection from infection) and platelets (for coagulation): it is sometimes caused by drugs: it is often fatal.

APPENDICITIS: inflammation of the appendix, the evolutionary remains of a part of the intestine important in herbivores.

APPETITE SUPPRESSANTS: drugs related to amphetamines reduce the usual readiness of dogs for food: they are used in the management of obesity: they have little effect and what they do have soon wears off, though they may help the weak-willed to make a start with self-control which is the only treatment for simple over-eating.

ARSPHENAMINE (SALVARSAN): the first product of a rational research programme to develop antibacterial chemotherapy: effective against syphilis: had serious adverse effects: an organic arsenic derivative.

ASPARAGINASE: a bacterial enzyme used in treatment of leukaemia.

ASPIRIN: acetylsalicylic acid: one of the first modern synthetic drugs: relieves pain, fever and inflammation probably by inhibiting the enzyme prostaglandin synthetase so that less inflammatory prostaglandin is released in response to tissue injury.

ASTHMA: an allergic disease characterized by contraction of the muscle, and so narrowing, of the bronchial tubes which conduct air to and from the gas exchanging alveoli of the lung: it causes difficulty in breathing.

ATROPINE: a substance found in the deadly nightshade plant (Atropa belladonna): it selectively blocks the effects of acetylcholine at some nerve endings: it is used by ophthalmologists to dilate the pupil of the eye and to paralyse its focusing to facilitate diagnostic examination: women used to employ it, despite the attendant disadvantages on focusing, to make their eyes seem dark, lustrous pools of sensuality.

BACTERIA: small unicellular organisms without a nucleus: some cause disease, some are useful, even essential, to man and some are merely indifferent.

BARBITURATE: a group of potent, sedative, hypnotic, antiepileptic and anaesthetic drugs developed in Germany: the parent compound (barbituric acid) was named after 'a charming lady named Barbara' of whom the synthesizer (1864) was enamoured: and the synthesizer (1903) of one of the most popular hypnotic derivatives (diethybarbituric acid) 'was struck with the idea of naming this compound Veronal' as he approached the city of Verona (Italy).[1]

BETA (β) – ADRENOCEPTORS: BETA-ADRENOCEPTOR BLOCKING DRUGS: a group of drugs that selectively blocks the beta rather than the alpha receptors responsive to adrenaline: used in heart disease and high blood pressure: commonly called 'beta-blockers': see adrenoceptors.

BIOAVAILABILITY: the amount of drug contained in a formulation, tablet, capsule, etc., that becomes available for absorption into the body.

BOTULINUM TOXIN: the poisonous substance (toxin) produced by a bacterium (Clostridium botulinum) causes paralysis by preventing the release of acetylcholine from nerve endings: grows in absence of air, e.g. in improperly canned food.

BRONCHI: tubes distributing air throughout the lungs.

BRONCHODILATION /BRONCHOCONSTRICTION: increased or decreased diameter of the bronchi due to relaxation or contraction of the muscular wall allowing freer or obstructed flow of air.

BUNSEN (BURNER): a gas/air jet heater used in laboratories: devised by R. W. E. van Bunsen (1811-99), Germany.

CACHET: a rice-paper container for a powder for swallowing.

CAFFEINE: the ingredient of coffee and tea that refreshes and keeps you awake.

CAPSULE: a soluble, e.g. gelatin, shell used to contain a dose of powdered drug.

CARBENOXOLONE (BIOGASTRONE): a derivative of liquorice that has a modest effect in promoting healing of peptic ulcer.

CARCINOGENESIS: causation of a malignant tumour (cancer).

CARDIAC: pertaining to the heart.

CARDIOVASCULAR SYSTEM: the heart and blood vessels (arteries, capillaries, veins).

[1] Miller, L. C. (1961), *Journal of the American Medical Association, 177*, 27.

CHEMOTHERAPY: the treatment of parasitic diseases (bacterial, protozoal) with drugs that do not harm the host: an example of selective toxicity.

CHIANTI: Italian wine from Tuscany.

CHLORAMPHENICOL (CHLOROMYCETIN): an antibiotic made by a mould (Streptomyces venezuelae): it has a wide range of anti-bacterial effects: rarely it causes aplastic anaemia, and since this is commonly fatal the use of the drug is restricted to serious conditions.

CHLOROFORM: the second (ether was the first) important volatile liquid general anaesthetic, introduced in 1847: can kill by depression of the heart and liver damage.

CHLOROQUINE (NIVAQUINE): an antimalarial drug found by chance to be beneficial also in resistant cases of rheumatoid arthritis: prolonged heavy dosage can damage the eye.

CHLORPROMAZINE (LARGACTIL): a major tranquillizer, particularly useful in schizophrenic states.

CHOLINESTERASE: enzyme that splits and so inactivates acetyl-choline.

CHRONIC: long continued: use of the word to mean 'disagreeable' is misuse.

CIMETIDINE (TAGAMET): a histamine H_2-receptor blocking drug: gastric acid is produced in response to the hormone gastrin which releases histamine which activates the H_2-receptor on the acid-secreting cell: cimetidine occupies this receptor without activating it: thus it prevents histamine from acting and producing acid: cimetidine increases healing of peptic ulcer.

CINCHONA BARK: from South America: contains the antimalarial quinine which is also used for its bitter flavour in 'tonic water' and aperitifs.

CLINICAL: pertaining to the sick bed: thus the practice of diagnostic and therapeutic medicine: the word is often misused to imply a detached coldness of manner.

CLIOQUINOL (ENTERO-VIOFORM): a weak antibacterial and amoebicide (amoebic dysentery) of dubious value and curious toxicity, particularly to the Japanese.

CODEINE: an active principle of opium used against cough and pain.

CONTRACEPTIVE: drug or appliance that prevents pregnancy.

CONVULSANT: causes convulsions.

CORNEA: the transparent front of the eye.

CORONARY THROMBOSIS: blood clot in artery supplying the heart muscle.

CRISIS: used in relation to fever it means the body temperature falls abruptly (crisis) rather than gradually (lysis).

CURARE: substance from South American plant that paralyses by selectively blocking acetylcholine receptors on voluntary muscle: arrow poison: victims die by paralysis of respiration and may safely be eaten since curare is not soluble in lipids and therefore does not enter the blood when swallowed.

DDT (DICOPHANE): insecticide: the most widely distributed man-made chemical in the world: probably no human being has none in his body: progressively being banned for fear of long-term adverse effects, but it has saved innumerable lives by killing malarial mosquitoes.

DEADLY NIGHTSHADE: Atropa belladonna, a plant containing atropine which selectively blocks some acetylcholine receptors.

DEPENDENCE: a condition in which an individual feels a need, psychological and/or physical, to continue to take a drug: if the drug is not available then 'withdrawal symptoms' occur: heroin and barbiturates are prominent examples as are alcohol and tobacco.

DIABETES MELLITUS: a disease due to lack of production of insulin in the body (juvenile-onset) or to resistance of the tissues to the action of insulin (maturity-onset).

DIARRHOEA: frequent and more or less fluid bowel motions.

DIGOXIN/DIGITOXIN: natural substances (glycosides) from foxglove species (Digitalis) used to strengthen the heart and regulate its rate and rhythm.

DIPHENOXYLATE + ATROPINE (LOMOTIL): an antidiarrhoea drug (diphenoxylate) combined with atropine to cause dry mouth so that the patient gets an early warning of overdose.

DIPHTHERIA: a serious infectious bacterial disease, usually affecting the throat: preventable by immunization.

DOPA: dihydroxyphenylalanine: a precursor of noradrenaline.

DRUG: defined by a World Health Organization Scientific Group as 'any substance or product that is used or intended to be used to modify or explore physiological systems or pathological states for the benefit of the recipient': pharmacologists widen the definition to include all substances that modify living tissue, thus including poisons: the use of the term to mean only substances subject to abuse as in 'you are not giving me a drug are you, doctor?', is deplorable.

DUODENUM: the part of the intestine leading out of the stomach: it receives the acid gastric contents.

ECZEMA: itching, inflammatory skin disease, sometimes an allergy.

ELECTROCARDIOGRAPH: record of the electrical activity of the heart muscle obtained from electrodes on the limbs and chest: useful in diagnosis of heart disease.

EMBOLISM: see thromboembolism.

ENDOCRINE GLAND/SECRETION: ductless glands make substances (hormones) that pass into the blood for carriage round the body, e.g. pituitary gland, adrenal gland, thyroid gland, ovary, testis.

ENDOMETRIUM/IAL: the lining of the uterus that is shed monthly in menstruation.

ENZYME: a catalytic substance, i.e. it facilitates chemical reactions without itself being altered so that it remains available continuously: living tissue depends on rapid chemical reactions: heat is the ordinary means of speeding up reactions: in living tissues the heat needed from external sources (sunlight) is insufficient and too irregular to allow continuous fast activity: enzymes do the job.

EPHEDRINE: an adrenaline-like substance obtained from a plant (Ephedra).

EPIDURAL ANAESTHESIA: passage of a fine tube into the lower end of the spinal canal through which a local anaesthetic is injected: this technique is used for pain-free labour: it is not free from complications.

EPILEPSY: a disease of recurrent convulsions: the commonest form is called idiopathic epilepsy because its cause is unknown.

EPINEPHRINE: synonym for adrenaline, which see.

ERGOMETRINE (ERGONOVINE): a derivative of a fungus (Claviceps purpurea) that grows on rye: it causes the uterus to contract and is used in obstetrics.

ERGOTAMINE/ERGOTOXINE: derivatives of ergot: the former is useful in migraine: the latter is a mixture of three substances.

ERGOT: a fungus growing on the cereal rye: it manufactures an extraordinary range of interesting substances, ergotamine, ergometrine, histamine, acetylcholine.

FIBRILLATION: unco-ordinated muscle contraction so that no useful work is done: can affect the different parts of the heart (atria, ventricles).

FORMALDEHYDE: a gas which in 37% solution in water is known as formalin: kills all living tissue.

FOXGLOVE: the Digitalis plants which provide glycosides that are useful in heart failure and disorders of cardiac rhythm.

FUNGUS/I: plants without chlorophyll so that they cannot synthesize organic substances and must therefore live on organic material, i.e. other plants and animals, dead or alive.

GALL STONES: stones formed in the bile, which is a fluid secreted by the liver and delivered by a network of passages into the small intestine where it assists the digestion of fats.

GANGLION-BLOCKING DRUGS: drugs which block the outlying relay station (ganglion) on the nerves controlling involuntary functions such as blood vessel diameter, intestinal movement, glandular secretion, etc.

GASTRIC: pertaining to the stomach.

GASTRIN: a hormone that is released into the blood when food is taken and that stimulates the stomach lining to secrete acid and digestive enzymes.

GENTAMICIN (GENTICIN): an antibiotic made by a mould Micromonospora purpurea.

GLANDULAR FEVER: infectious mononucleosis: an infective virus disease affecting lymphoid tissues of the body concerned with immunity: curiously, if a patient is given ampicillin (one of the semi-synthetic penicillins) a skin rash almost always follows.

GLAUCOMA: a condition in which the pressure within the eye increases: if untreated it can cause blindness.

GONORRHOEA: a bacterial infection chiefly affecting the urinary passages transmitted by sexual intercourse (venereal disease).

GOUT: an extremely painful condition due to formation of crystals of urate in the tissues, particularly the joints: see probenecid and allopurinol.

HAEMOLYSIS: destruction of red blood cells inside the circulation.

HALOTHANE (FLUOTHANE): a general anaesthetic: repeated use can rarely cause liver damage.

HAEMORRHAGE/HAGIC: bleeding.

HAY-FEVER (ALLERGIC RHINITIS): a recurrent seasonal pollen allergy affecting the eye and nasal passages and characterized by itching, watery discharge and sneezing.

HEARTBURN: a painful sensation experienced in the lower centre of the chest due to reflux of stomach acid into the oesophagus (gullet): nothing at all to do with the heart.

HERNIA: the intestine bulges through a weak area of the abdominal wall, commonly in the groin.

HEROIN: diacetylmorphine: a semi-synthetic morphine derivative: can be made in a kitchen: a potent analgesic: has been much abused and so is illegal even in medicine in many countries, e.g. USA: still available in medicine in UK.

HISTAMINE: a biologically active substance playing a part in allergic reactions and gastric acid secretion: there are two types of receptor, H_1 and H_2.

HOMOEOPATHY: system of medicine founded on the belief that drugs that in large doses cause certain symptoms will, in small doses, cure similar symptoms when these are due to disease: a scientifically dubious proposition: the classic work that expounds the system is Samuel Hahnemann's *Organon of the*

Rational Art of Healing (1810).

HORMONE: chemical messenger: chemical regulator produced by specialized cells that is transported round the body by the blood to affect cells remote from its origin, e.g. insulin, gastrin.

HYPERTENSION: high blood pressure.

HYPNOTIC: a drug that promotes sleep.

HYPOGLYCAEMIA: low blood sugar concentration causing illness.

IMIPRAMINE (TOFRANIL): an antidepressant drug.

INFECTION: growth of another organism, whether bacterium, virus, fungus, protozoan (unicellular animal) etc., within the body so as to cause disease.

INSULIN: a hormone of the pancreatic gland that regulates glucose metabolism and therefore energy production: its absence is a cause of diabetes mellitus.

INTRACRANIAL: inside the skull.

IONIZATION: the process of producing ions, i.e. atoms or groups of atoms which have lost or gained one electron: the process causes important changes in physico-chemical properties of drugs, particularly affecting solubility in lipids and as a result, the property of diffusing across cellular boundaries in the body.

ISONIAZID (RIMIFON): an antituberculosis drug.

KIDNEY: the kidney may be regarded as a filter for the blood: water and all molecules smaller than protein are filtered out unselectively into a system of small tubes from which the kidney then reabsorbs what is necessary to maintain the body in health, the rest being eliminated as urine: the kidney provides a major route of elimination of drugs.

LIGNOCAINE (XYLOCAINE): a local anaesthetic drug.

LINIMENT: a liquid for rubbing into the skin: usually contains irritant substances that cause locally increased blood flow and a feeling of warmth: comforting, especially if it smells strongly: effect largely as placebo.

LIPOPROTEIN: substances consisting of a combination of fat with protein: animal cell walls consist of lipoprotein.

LOTION: a solution in water for local application, e.g. skin, eye.

LOZENGE: a formulation of a drug for sucking.

LYSERGIC ACID DIETHYLAMIDE/LSD_{25}: lysergic acid is a substance found in ergot: the famous hallucinogen LSD_{25} is a semisynthetic derivative the effect of which was discovered by accident in the research department of a Swiss drug company.

MACROMOLECULE: big molecule.

MALARIA: infection by a unicellular organism (Plasmodium) causing recurrent fever: transmitted by mosquito bites.

MALATHION: an insecticide that acts by inhibiting (blocking) the enzyme cholinesterase.

MASTITIS: inflammation of the female breast or udder.

MASTOID: the bulge of bone behind the ear (mastoid process) of cellular structure and prone to infection along with the middle ear: infection can extend into the skull and cause meningitis: in chronic cases surgery was employed to eliminate the infection: with modern antibiotics this is now rarely necessary.

MEDICINE: a formulation of a drug or drugs into a suitable form for administration in the treatment of disease by any route, e.g. by mouth, by injection, on the skin, etc.

MENINGITIS: inflammation of the membranes surrounding the brain and spinal cord: usually bacterial: a serious disease.

MEPACRINE: one of the first synthetic antimalarial drugs.

METABOLISM: the process of synthesizing or breaking down foods and drugs.

METHYLDOPA (ALDOMET): a drug useful in treating high blood pressure.

MONOAMINE OXIDASE: an enzyme that inactivates monoamines such as tyramine formed in cheese, which substance, if not inactivated in the gut wall, enters the circulation and causes high blood pressure by releasing noradrenaline from storage sites in nerve endings on blood vessels.

MORPHINE: principal active analgesic in opium: can easily be made into heroin.

MUCOSA/MUCOUS MEMBRANE: a membrane lining a body passage or cavity that contains mucus-secreting cells: mucus gives a protective lubricant coating, e.g. saliva.

MULTIPLE SCLEROSIS: a disease of unknown cause characterized by recurrent attacks of localized inflammation in the brain and spinal cord.

MUTAGENESIS: causation of genetic change which can be transmitted by cell division.

MYASTHENIA GRAVIS: condition in which there is muscle weakness, especially with repeated movement (fatiguability) due to a defect of the nerve-muscle junction.

MYOCARDIAL INFARCTION: the heart muscle (myocardium) is damaged by blocking of a blood vessel so that it dies: depending on the size of vessel blocked the area of muscle damage may be small or large.

NEOARSPHENAMINE (NEOSALVARSAN): an effective agent against syphilis, a superior substitute for arsphenamine, which see.

NEOSTIGMINE (PROSTIGMIN): a drug that blocks the enzyme cholinesterase that breaks down the chemical (acetylcholine) that transmits the nerve impulse to the muscles: an anticholinesterase drug.

NEPHROPATHY: damage/disease of the kidney.

NICOTINE: the principal active substance in tobacco: it has highly specific actions on nervous tissue: an 'enjoyment poison' (Genussgift).

NITRATES: various nitrates, e.g. glyceryl trinitrate, are useful to relieve or prevent the pain of angina pectoris.

NORADRENALINE: the principal chemical transmitter released at some involuntary (sympathetic) nerve endings: it activates receptors on involuntary muscle, bronchi, blood vessels, heart.

NOREPINEPHRINE: synonym for noradrenaline, which see.

OESTRADIOL: a female sex hormone.

OESTROGENS: the female sex hormones.

OINTMENT: a semi-solid preparation for local application, e.g. skin, eye.

OPIATE: drug derived from opium, which is the dried juice of the oriental poppy (Papaver somniferum): the chief opiate is morphine.

OPIUM: dried juice of the opium poppy (Papaver somniferum) contains morphine and codeine.

OXYTOCIN: a hormone of the posterior pituitary gland: it is largely responsible for uterine contractions in labour: it is now made synthetically and is available for use in obstetrics.

PAMAQUIN: a synthetic antimalarial drug.

PARACETAMOL (PANADOL): a minor analgesic sold directly to the public for aches and pains: overdose can cause liver damage and death.

PANDEMIC: prevalent all over the world.

PARASITE: an organism living on another and drawing nourishment directly from it: bacteria, fungi and worms are all parasites producing disease in man.

PENICILLIN: an antibiotic originally obtained from a mould Penicillium notatum: synthetic chemists have now modified the molecule to provide a range of penicillins of varying antibacterial range: this is an example of useful 'molecular manipulation'.

PEPTIC ULCER: ulcer of the stomach and duodenum (the part of the small intestine leading from the stomach and receiving the acid gastric juice).

PERIPHERAL NEURITIS: inflammation of the nerves leaving the brain and spinal cord to supply outlying organs, muscles, skin, etc.: weakness and loss of sensation occur.

PERITONITIS/(PERITONEAL): inflammation of the smooth mucosal membrane lining the abdominal cavity and that allows the intestines freedom to change size and to move as the food within them is propelled onwards by muscular contractions.

PERNICIOUS ANAEMIA: disease due to failure of the stomach lining to make substance necessary for the body to absorb vitamin B_{12} from the food.

PESSARY: a formulation for administration of a drug via the vagina.

pH: symbol used to express hydrogen ion concentration: acid solutions liberate hydrogen ions: alkaline solutions liberate hydroxyl ions: this expresses acidity and alkalinity.

PHARMACOPOEIA: a book listing drugs with standards of purity, formulation and directions for use: in many countries there is an official pharmacopoeia setting legally enforceable standards.

PHENACETIN: a minor analgesic generally in a combined tablet with aspirin and codeine or caffeine: prolonged heavy dosage can damage the kidney.

PHENAZONE: an obsolescent/obsolete minor analgesic prone to cause skin rashes.

PHENOBARBITONE: a member of the barbiturate (which see) series of drugs: effective against epilepsy unlike other barbiturates.

PHENOL: carbolic acid: a potent antiseptic obtained from coal tar: kills all living tissue.

PHENOTHIAZINE TRANQUILLIZERS: the first major tranquillizers producing significant benefit in schizophrenia.

PHENYLBUTAZONE (BUTAZOLIDIN): an anti-inflammation drug used in rheumatism and arthritis: can cause agranulocytosis and gastric bleeding.

PHEROMONES: hormones released by animals to obtain response from other animals of the same species, e.g. a mated female mouse fails to become pregnant if exposed to the smell of an alien male: sexual attraction in moths, often over enormous distances.

PHOCOMELIA: limbs like those of a seal, i.e. short upper and lower sections of the limb so that hand and foot seem to arise directly from the body: the characteristic fetal deformity produced by thalidomide.

PITUITARY GLAND: situated at the base of the brain it produces a variety of hormones and has been described as the 'conductor of the endocrine orchestra', i.e. some of its hormones control other ductless (hormone-producing) glands.

PLACEBO: a medicine given to please the recipient but having no pharmacological beneficial effect: tonics are placebos.

PLASMA: the liquid (non-cellular) phase of the blood.

PLASMA PROTEINS: protein in the liquid (non-cellular) phase of the blood: various natural substances and drugs are carried attached to plasma proteins and may displace each other causing, for example, interesting drug interactions.

PNEUMONIA: inflammation of the lung usually due to bacteria or virus: it may be patchy or diffuse throughout the lung or affect one of the anatomical lobes (lobar pneumonia).

POLYPEPTIDE: a substance consisting of a string of amino acids linked by their amino and carboxyl groups.

POST-MORTEM: after death.

PRACTOLOL (ERALDIN): a beta-adrenoceptor blocking drug having a selective action on the heart (so it did not make asthma worse as do unselective drugs of this group): used in angina pectoris and high blood pressure: abandoned after it was found to damage the eyes, etc.

PRIMAQUINE: an antimalarial.

PROBENECID (BENEMID): a drug that blocks the active transport of acid substances across the walls of the small tubes in the kidney with the result that it prevents the elimination of penicillin (an acid) by the kidney and also prevents the re-absorption back into the blood of uric acid that has been filtered out of the blood: the drug is thus used to enhance the blood levels of penicillin and to prevent gout.

PROGESTOGEN: a female sex hormone.

PROGNOSIS: forecast of the outcome or future course of disease.

PRONETHALOL: the first beta-adrenoceptor blocking drug used (in angina pectoris): abandoned after it was suspected of causing cancer in mice.

PROPRANOLOL (INDERAL): a beta-adrenoceptor blocking drug.

PROSTAGLANDINS: aliphatic acids: substances released in the body as part of the inflammatory response: possible other functions as chemical transmitters in the brain: thought to have been first observed in the secretion of the male prostate gland, though this was an error because they were in a seminal vesicle secretion: an example of the inadvisability of giving substances names based on assumed origin or function.

PROSTAGLANDIN SYNTHETASE: an enzyme that catalyses the synthesis of prostaglandins: the benefit of aspirin and other anti-inflammatory drugs may be due to inhibition of this enzyme.

PROTEINS: complex substances characteristic of living matter: they are made up of amino acids.

PROTOZOA: small unicellular organisms having a nucleus (unlike bacteria).

PSORIASIS: a disfiguring scaly skin disease.

PSYCHOSOMATIC ILLNESS: an illness of the body wholly or partly caused by mental stress or illness.

PSYCHOTROPIC: alters brain/mind function.

PURGATIVE: drug that causes bowel evacuation: much domestic

use of these drugs is unnecessary.

PUS: yellowish fluid product of bacterial infection: consists largely of white blood cells that have died in battle.

PYOGENIC: pus producing: pus is largely white blood cells that have died defending the body against invading bacteria.

QUININE: antimalarial drug: occurs in cinchona bark from South America.

RECEPTORS: specialized molecules on cell surface that recognize/interact with specific chemicals that fit them alone: receptors are a means by which chemical messengers in the body as well as drugs produce selective effects.

RESERPINE: a pure substance obtained from an Indian plant, Rauwolfia serpentina, obsolescent as a tranquillizer, but still used in high blood pressure: can cause serious mental depression.

RETINA: the light-sensitive tissue at the back of the eye on which the lens focuses the image.

RHEUMATOID ARTHRITIS: a chronic inflammation of the joints chiefly of those farthest from the trunk: of uncertain cause.

RIGOR: attack of shivering usually due to an infection.

SALBUTAMOL (VENTOLIN): a selective activator of beta-adreno-ceptors on bronchial muscle: valuable in asthma.

SEDATIVE: a drug that quietens without causing sleep.

SEPSIS: bacterial infection.

SEPTICAEMIA: a serious condition in which bacteria grow in the blood stream: 'mere presence of bacteria in the blood is called bacteraemia.

SODIUM CROMOGLYCATE (INTAL): drug used in allergy such as asthma and hay-fever to prevent the antigen/antibody reaction from causing release from cells of histamine and other active substances which cause bronchoconstriction.

SODIUM VALPROATE (EPILIM): an antiepileptic drug.

SPIROCHAETE: causative organism of syphilis.

STAPHYLOCOCCUS/I: bacteria that cause boils, abscesses and a variety of serious infections: some of them are resistant to penicillin because they are able to destroy the drug by making an enzyme, penicillinase.

STREPTOCOCCUS/I: bacteria that cause sore throats and a variety of serious infections.

STREPTOMYCIN: an antibiotic from a mould Streptomyces griseus: the first successful antituberculosis drug.

STRYCHNINE: a powerful convulsion-producing substance from the plant genus Strychnos: obsolete in medicine (as a tonic): rarely used to poison vermin because of hazard to man and

the animals he does not wish to kill: also, there are less unpleasant alternatives.

SUCCINYLCHOLINE (SCOLINE): briefly blocks the transmission of the
nerve impulse to voluntary muscle, thus paralysing the patient:
used to provide muscular relaxation for anaesthetic and surgical
procedures.

SULPHONAMIDES: the first synthetic drugs effective against common bacterial infections.

SUPPOSITORY: a formulation for administration of a drug via the
anus: a substantial proportion, a survey has revealed, are
inserted by the patient without prior removal of the wrapper.

SYMBIOSIS: two organisms living attached to each other to mutual
advantage, e.g. some bacteria in the human intestine manufacture vitamin K, essential for adequate blood coagulation.

SYMPATHETIC NERVES: sympathetic nervous system: part of the
involuntary or automatic (autonomic) nervous system that controls activity of the heart, blood vessels, bronchi, intestines, etc.:
the transmitter at the nerve endings is noradrenaline.

SYMPATHOLYTIC: reducing the activity of the sympathetic nervous
system.

SYMPATHOMIMETIC: mimicking the effects of, or activating, the
sympathetic nervous system.

SYPHILIS: a sexually transmitted disease with severe long-term
effects on the central nervous and cardiovascular systems: it
can affect the fetus.

TABLET: a solid drug dose form made by compression.

TERATOGENESIS: causation of an abnormality of the fetus.

TETANUS TOXIN: the poisonous substance produced by the tetanus
bacillus which causes convulsions: the bacillus lives in the soil
and in faeces: tetanus is an unpleasant and often fatal disease:
effective immunization is available.

TETRACYCLINES: antibiotics made from moulds, Streptomyces
aureofaciens and rimosus: semi-synthetic variants are in use.

THALIDOMIDE: the notorious hypnotic drug that causes grave fetal
abnormalities, particularly affecting the limbs.

THERAPY/THERAPEUTIC: treatment of disease: the sometimes seen
expression 'therapeutic treatment' is a tautology.

THIAZIDE: a group of diuretic drugs, which eliminate, via the
urine, fluid retained in the body as in heart failure: also
effective against high blood pressure.

THROMBOEMBOLISM: blood clot inside a vessel (thrombosis) breaks
free, floats along until it plugs a small vessel: a common
example is a clot from a vein in the leg passing up through
the heart and ending its journey in the lung (pulmonary
embolism): always a serious condition.

THROMBOSIS: clotting of blood in a vessel so as to narrow or block it.

THYROID GLAND: an endocrine organ whose hormones, thyroxine and triiodothyronine control growth, metabolism and differentiation.

TONIC: a placebo.

TRANQUILLIZER: a drug that quietens mental agitation without inducing sleep: this is not as clear a distinction as it may sound, in high doses tranquillizers can induce sleep, and there are some drugs that only tranquillize at the cost of considerable drowsiness.

TRYPANOSOMES/TRYPANOSOMIASIS: a single-cell (protozoal) organism that causes tropical sleeping sickness, spread by the tsetse fly.

TUBERCULOSIS: infection by Mycobacterium tuberculosis: most common in the lungs, but can affect any tissue.

TYRAMINE: a monoamine formed from the amino acid tyrosine by bacteria in cheese or other food: it is normally inactivated in the gut wall by the protective enzyme monoamine oxidase so that it does not enter the body: if the enzyme is blocked by a monoamine oxidase inhibitor (used against depression) then tyramine enters the body and causes high blood pressure: such patients have died of brain haemorrhage after eating cheese.

ULCER/GASTRIC/DUODENAL: see peptic ulcer.

URIC ACID: synthesized in the body from purine precursors, xanthine and hypoxanthine: a high concentration of uric acid (as urate) leads to the formation of urate crystals in the tissues, particularly of the joints: this is gout, a very painful condition.

UTOPIA: title of a book published in 1516 by Sir Thomas More, about an imaginary place with a perfect social and political system.

VASODILATOR: dilates blood vessels, increasing blood flow to a part of the body and lowering blood pressure.

VENEREAL: relating to sexual intercourse.

VIRUS: a simple organism, smaller than bacteria, capable only of existing in living cells: a non-living nucleic acid particle, usually encapsulated in protein, a virus multiplies at the expense of cells that it infects.

VITAMIN: an accessory food factor present in many foods and essential to health: only small amounts are needed: lack of vitamin C causes scurvy, of vitamin D causes rickets.

VITAMIN B_{12}: essential for forming red blood cells: deficiency causes pernicious anaemia.

Index

Technosphere

Technosphere is an original Fontana series that presents individual studies of particular sciences and technologies in terms of their human repercussions. The series will include original analyses of a wide variety of subjects – transport technology, drugs, computer technology, operational research and systems analysis, photography, urban planning, films, alternative medicine, and so on – with the emphasis on the present state of the science or technology in question, its social significance, and the future direction of its probable and necessary development.

Technosphere is edited by Jonathan Benthall, Director of the Royal Anthropological Institute.

Already published:

Television: Technology and Culutral Form
by Raymond Williams

Through a survey of the development of television and broadcasting institutions in Britain and America, and an analysis of the different programming forms and their scheduling by the BBC, ITV and American networks, Raymond Williams seriously questions current views on television, and maps out a critical approach to programmes as varied as 'Coronation Street' and 'News at Ten'. '. . . a powerful and reasoned attack on technological determinism.'   Stuart Hood, *Guardian*

Alternative Technology and the Politics of Technical Change
by David Dickson

David Dickson's searching analysis clearly demonstrates that, as man is forced by increasing scarcity to consume less at a time when he is compelled by economic necessity to produce more, so he must adopt fresh attitudes to technology. The characteristics of these fresh attitudes are outlined in terms that are clear and positive but reflect the tentative and experimental character of all alternative technology.

'. . . entirely convincing . . . Dickson's statement of the case for the non-neutrality of technology is by far the best I have come across.'
New Society

An Open University set book

Fontana Books

Fontana is a leading paperback publisher of fiction and non-fiction, with authors ranging from Alistair MacLean, Agatha Christie and Desmond Bagley to Solzhenitsyn and Pasternak, from Gerald Durrell and Joy Adamson to the famous Modern Masters series.

In addition to a wide-ranging collection of internationally popular writers of fiction, Fontana also has an outstanding reputation for history, natural history, military history, psychology, psychiatry, politics, economics, religion and the social sciences.

All Fontana books are available at your bookshop or newsagent; or can be ordered direct. Just fill in the form and list the titles you want.
